Fluoro-Flip
A Quick Reference Guide to Spinal and Peripheral Pain Procedures

Fluoro-Flip
A Quick Reference Guide to Spinal and Peripheral Pain Procedures

Rudy Garza III MD
Interventional Pain Medicine Physician
Department of Anesthesiology and Pain Medicine
Clinical Assistant Professor
UT Health San Antonio
San Antonio, Texas, USA
Proudly serving the community of Bexar County and the surrounding counties

Co-Authors

Maxim S Eckmann MD
Medical Director of Pain Medicine
Program Director, UT Health Pain Medicine Fellowship
Director, Translational Research
Associate Professor
UT Health San Antonio
San Antonio, Texas, USA

Rachel Yinfei Xu MD
Physical Medicine and Interventional Pain Medicine Physician
Private Practice
San Antonio, Texas, USA

Foreword

Maxim S Eckmann MD

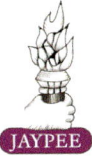

JAYPEE BROTHERS MEDICAL PUBLISHERS
The Health Sciences Publisher
New Delhi | London

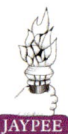

Jaypee Brothers Medical Publishers (P) Ltd

Headquarters
EMCA House
23/23-B, Ansari Road, Daryaganj
New Delhi 110 002, India
Landline: +91-11-23272143, +91-11-23272703
+91-11-23282021, +91-11-23245672
E-mail: jaypee@jaypeebrothers.com

Overseas Office
J.P. Medical Ltd.
83, Victoria Street, London
SW1H 0HW (UK)
Phone: +44-20 3170 8910
E-mail: info@jpmedpub.com

Corporate Office
4838/24, Ansari Road, Daryaganj
New Delhi 110 002, India
Phone: +91-11-43574357
Fax: +91-11-43574314
E-mail: jaypee@jaypeebrothers.com

EU GPSR Authorised Representative
Logos Europe, 9 rue Nicolas Poussin
17000, La Rochelle, France
Phone: +33 (0) 6 67 93 73 78
E-mail: contact@logoseurope.eu

Website: www.jaypeebrothers.com
Website: www.jaypeedigital.com

© **2018, Jaypee Brothers Medical Publishers**

The views and opinions expressed in this book are solely those of the original contributor(s)/author(s) and do not necessarily represent those of editor(s) of the book.

All rights reserved. No part of this publication may be reproduced, stored or transmitted in any form or by any means, electronic, mechanical, photocopying, recording or otherwise, without the prior permission in writing of the publishers.

All brand names and product names used in this book are trade names, service marks, trademarks or registered trademarks of their respective owners. The publisher is not associated with any product or vendor mentioned in this book.

Medical knowledge and practice change constantly. This book is designed to provide accurate, authoritative information about the subject matter in question. However, readers are advised to check the most current information available on procedures included and check information from the manufacturer of each product to be administered, to verify the recommended dose, formula, method and duration of administration, adverse effects and contraindications. It is the responsibility of the practitioner to take all appropriate safety precautions. Neither the publisher nor the author(s)/editor(s) assume any liability for any injury and/or damage to persons or property arising from or related to use of material in this book.

This book is sold on the understanding that the publisher is not engaged in providing professional medical services. If such advice or services are required, the services of a competent medical professional should be sought.

Every effort has been made where necessary to contact holders of copyright to obtain permission to reproduce copyright material. If any have been inadvertently overlooked, the publisher will be pleased to make the necessary arrangements at the first opportunity. The **CD/DVD-ROM** (if any) provided in the sealed envelope with this book is complimentary and free of cost. **Not meant for sale.**

Inquiries for bulk sales may be solicited at: jaypee@jaypeebrothers.com

Fluoro-Flip: A Quick Reference Guide to Spinal and Peripheral Pain Procedures
First Edition: 2018, *Reprint:* 2026

ISBN: 978-93-5270-302-9

Printed in India

Dedication

"I am not what you would call a handsome man. The good Lord chose not to bless me with ... with charm, athletic ability...or a fully functional brain." — *Paco (WaterBoy)*

But what he did bless me with are three beautiful children Brandon, Dylan, and Nicholas and a loving and supportive wife. Without you Veronica, my dreams would always be dreams and would never become reality.

Foreword

As a Pain Fellowship Program Director, I have had the privilege and enjoyment of helping guide bright young minds in our field. I have similarly enjoyed learning from my colleagues and sharing my own knowledge with them at national and international training courses. If there is one resounding theme that I can echo with Dr Rudy Garza, it is that the safe and effective performance of interventional pain procedures presents a steep learning curve that continues beyond residency and fellowship training.

"The five-Stage Model of Adult Skill Acquisition", as described by the esteemed Professor Stuart E Dreyfus, outlines the evolution of learning at an advanced level—as physicians must continually do in an era of constant technological advancement. We all start as Novices, regardless of innate intelligence, and move on to stages of Advanced Beginner, Competence, Proficiency, and Expertise. We would all strive to reach Expert level, thereby being able to see "what needs to be achieved; thanks to his or her vast repertoire of situational discriminations", and immediately (instinctively) understand how to achieve this goal. However, the cognitive complexities of understanding human anatomy, interpreting imaging, overcoming adverse conditions—in the setting of battling provider fatigue and time demands—makes attaining "Expert" status a lofty but difficult goal.

In reflecting on my own practice, I can say that there are domains in which I feel I am an Expert after about a decade of practice in advanced pain interventions, yet also domains that I am newly exploring and having to process at a more novice level. While some knowledge translates and facilitates adopting new techniques, I find that there is no replacement for hands-on, real-time experience. I acknowledge that attaining new skills is a daunting and sometimes frightening task, especially when one moves "away from the nest" of fellowship colleagues.

Our hope is that *Fluoro-Flip: A Quick Reference Guide to Spinal and Peripheral Pain Procedures*, can be a resource that facilitates advanced learning while providing comfort to the interventionist, who like most of us, is appropriately anxious when performing these important but potentially dangerous procedures. Serving as a low-tech time machine, "Fluoro-Flip" can take you back in time to when your own professor was showing you how to do a Gasserian Ganglion Block at the base of the skull, or take you forward in time to a more efficient pace with a well trained eye and informed fluoroscopy technician. Additionally, "Fluoro-Flip" can be a trusted companion when you need that quick "curbside" consult in the present moment.

While this resource is not intended to be a replacement for proper training, board certification, or experience, we believe it can assist the interventionist in being more confident with these image-guided pain procedures.

Maxim S Eckmann MD
Medical Director of Pain Medicine
Program Director
UT Health Pain Medicine Fellowship
Director
Translational Research
Associate Professor
UT Health San Antonio
San Antonio, Texas, USA

Preface

During my training, I had performed over six hundred fluoroscopic procedures, went to the best pain fellowship, and trained under one of the grandfathers of pain. I felt that I could tackle any procedure that was thrown at me. I graduated, and my confidence lasted all but a day. I no longer had someone holding me by the hand, getting the view, and telling me to "Light at the center of the hub!" Like most, I was under the assumption that once I go to private practice, I will have an X-ray technique that will line up the picture and it would be easy. Well I was wrong. So, instead of learning about the day-to-day operations of a practice, I focused my time on truly learning fluoroscopy. I went old school and pulled out Netter's, exposed patients to probably a year's worth of radiation and had countless conversations about techniques with my mentors and fellow colleagues. Overtime, I developed methods that helped me successfully perform blocks safely and efficiently.

There are many great books out there for spinal procedure, but limited resources on other peripheral blocks. This book is designed to serve as a radiographic guide to spinal, head and neck and peripheral blocks. I tried to simplify the procedures so that even the most novice practitioner, X-ray technician, or medical assistant can use this book and easily obtain the pictures to assist in performing the block. Each image has a side by side duplicate with landmarks and targets drawn out to assist in navigating through each block.

If anyone has suggestions for improvements or wants me to add other information, please email me at *fluoroflip@gmail.com*.
Thanks for reading.

Rudy Garza III MD

Acknowledgments

I cannot express enough the appreciation I have for my pain "brothren" for their support and encouragement throughout my medical career: Dr Eckmann, Dr Nagpal, Dr Boies, Dr Mitchell, Dr Patel, and my fellowship classmates. You all have always been supportive to my ideas no matter how ridiculous they may have seemed. I especially would like to acknowledge Dr Ramamurthy for not only the learning opportunities he provided during my training but also his contributions to the field of Anesthesiology and Pain Medicine. I will forever model my practice as to "What would Dr Rama do?"

To Brandon, Dylan, and Nicholas—thank you for allowing me the time away from home to write this book. I am finally coming home at a scheduled time. You boys deserve a trip to the Bahamas!... but after football season of course.

To my caring, loving, and supportive wife, Veronica: my deepest gratitude. You are what keeps this boat afloat. I could not have asked for a better partner to share this life with.

I am also thankful to Mr Jitendar P Vij (Group Chairman), Mr Ankit Vij (Group President), Ms Chetna Malhotra Vohra (Associate Director-Content Strategy), and Ms Nedup Denka Bhutia (Development Editor) of Jaypee Brothers Medical Publishers, New Delhi, India, for giving me a go-ahead at the very beginning and helping me in every way possible to bring out this book.

Contents

1. **Basics to Fluoroscopy**   1
   - C-Arm *1*
   - Standard Set up *2*
   - Pain Procedure Current Procedure Terminology Codes (2017) *4*
   - Target Angles *6*

2. **Pharmacology**   9
   - Anticoagulation Guidelines *9*
   - Local Anesthetics *10*
   - Steroids *11*
   - Contrast Agents *12*

3. **Head, Neck and Upper Extremity**   15
   - Gasserian Ganglion Block *15*
   - Maxillary and Mandibular Nerve Block *18*
   - Sphenopalatine Ganglion Block *19*
   - Glossopharyngeal Nerve Block *20*
   - Cervical Facet Intra-articular Injection *22*
   - Atlantoaxial Intra-articular Injection *24*
   - Cervical Medial Branch Blocks and Radiofrequency Ablation *25*
   - Cervical Epidural Steroid Injection (Parasagittal Approach) *28*
   - Cervical Transforaminal Epidural Steroid Injection *30*
   - Spinal Cord Stimulator Trial—Cervical *32*
   - Stellate Ganglion Block *34*
   - Glenohumeral Shoulder Intra-articular Injection (Anterior Approach) *35*

4. Thoracic, Chest and Abdomen — 38

- Thoracic Intra-articular Facet Injection *38*
- Thoracic Medial Branch Block and Radiofrequency Ablation *40*
- Thoracic Epidural Steroid Injection (Parasagittal Approach) *42*
- Intercostal Nerve Blocks *44*
- Splanchnic Nerve Block (Retrocrural Technique) *45*
- Celiac Plexus Block (Transcrural Technique) *47*

5. Pelvis, Rectum and Perineum — 50

- Superior Hypogastric Plexus Block: Posterior Approach *50*
- Ganglion Impar Block: Sacrococcygeal/Intercoccygeal Joint Approach *52*
- Pudendal Nerve Block *54*

6. Lumbar Spine, Hips and Lower Extremities — 56

- Lumbar Interlaminar Epidural Steroid Injection: Parasagittal Approach *56*
- Lumbar Transforaminal Epidural Steroid Injection: Subpedicular Approach *58*
- Lumbar Transforaminal Epidural Steroid Injection: Supraneural Approach *60*
- Lumbar Transforaminal Epidural Steroid Injection: Retroneural Approach *62*
- Lumbar Transforaminal Epidural Steroid Injection: Infraneural Approach (Kambin's Triangle) *63*
- Caudal Epidural Steroid Injection *64*
- Lumbar Intra-articular Facet Joint Injection *66*
- Lumbar Medial Branch Block and Radiofrequency Ablation *68*
- Provocative Lumbar Discography *71*
- Spinal Cord Stimulator Trial—Lumbar *73*
- Intrathecal Trial—Lumbar *76*
- Sacroiliac Joint Injection: Inferior Approach *78*
- Dorsal Rami (L5) and Lateral Branch Blocks (S1-S3) *80*
- Lumbar Sympathetic Block *82*
- Intra-articular Hip Injection *82*
- Articular Branch Blocks of the Femoral and Obturator Nerves *84*
- Intra-articular Knee Injection *85*
- Knee Genicular Nerve Blocks (Four Locations) *86*

Index *91*

Terms/Abbreviations

- AP: Anteroposterior
- C1–C7: Cervical levels
- CESI: Cervical epidural steroid injection
- C MBB: Cervical medial branch block
- CRPS: Complex regional pain syndrome
- DR: Dorsal rami
- DRB: Dorsal ramus block
- DSA: Digital subtraction angiography
- ESI: Epidural steroid injection
- IAP: Inferior articular process
- L1–L5: Lumbar levels
- LBB: Lateral branch block
- LESI: Lumbar epidural steroid injection
- LM: Lateral mass
- L MBB: Lumbar medial branch block
- LOR: Loss of resistance
- MB: Medial branch
- MBB: Medial branch block
- NF: Neuroforamen
- PA: Posteroanterior
- PDPH: Post dural puncture headache
- PED: Pedicle
- PFNS: Preservative free normal saline
- RFA: Radiofrequency ablation
- S1–S5: Sacral levels
- SAP: Superior articular process
- SCS: Spinal cord stimulator
- SIJ: Sacroiliac joint
- SNRB: Selective nerve root block
- SP: Spinous process
- T1–T12: Thoracic levels
- TESI: Thoracic epidural steroid injection

- TFESI: Transforaminal epidural steroid injection
- TMBB: Thoracic medial branch block
- TON: Third occipital nerve
- TP: Transverse process
- UP: Uncinate process
- VB: Vertebral body

Chapter 1

Basics to Fluoroscopy

C-ARM

Components of the fluoroscopic imaging chain (Figs. 1.1 and 1.2):

X-ray generator: The X-ray generator delivers the electrical power to energize the X-ray tube and permits the selection of X-ray energy, X-ray quantity, and exposure time.

X-ray tube: It converts electrical energy from the X-ray generator to a X-ray beam. It is the source of radiation.

Collimator: It contains shutter blades that define the shape of the X-ray beam. Collimating the beam, or "coning down", results in less scatter X-ray beams and therefore a sharper image. It also reduces the overall radiation dose.

Patient table and pad: It is usually made from a carbon fiber composite material to minimize X-ray attenuation. Thin foam pads are better than thick gel pads.

Image intensifier: It converts the X-ray spectrum transmitted through the patient into a highly visible image and amplifies image brightness.

C-arm Maneuvers

Tilt versus Oblique Rotation
- All movements of the C-arm are in relation to the *image intensifier*.
  ◊ *Cephalad/cephalic tilt*: >C-arm angled to the patient's head
  ◊ *Caudate/caudal tilt*: >C-arm angled to the patient's feet

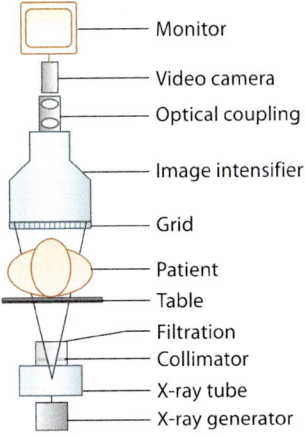

Fig. 1.1: Components of the fluoroscopic imaging chain.[1]

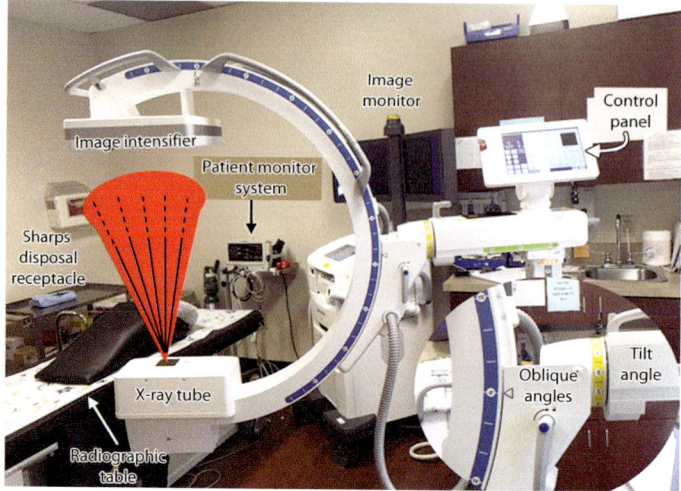

Fig. 1.2: The C-arm. The tube emits X-rays beams that penetrate the patient's body. The image intensifier converts the X-rays into a visible image that is then displayed on the image monitor. Distance, time, and shielding are the three most important basic guides for radiation safety. Radiation dose varies inversely to the square of the distance from the source. Always take a step back before you take a shot.

- ◊ *Ipsilateral oblique rotation*: >C-arm rotated toward the side of the injection
- ◊ *Contralateral oblique rotation*: >C-arm rotated toward the opposite side of the injection.

Anteroposterior versus Lateral
- *Anteroposterior (AP) view (different at each level based upon positioning, scoliosis, lordosis, etc.)*:
  - ◊ The spinous process is equidistant from both the pedicles
  - ◊ The vertebral body endplates are horizontal lines and not oval-shaped
  - ◊ AP versus PA (posteroanterior): Based upon X-ray tube. Using a C-arm, AP view are obtained when a patient is in the prone position (patient laying on the abdomen) versus PA view patients are supine (patient on their back).
  - ◊ Not necessarily at 0° from angulation.
- *Lateral view*:
  - ◊ Oblique 90° from a true AP view.

STANDARD SET UP (FIG. 1.3)
- Sterile gloves, mask, and scrub cap
- One Prep tray
- Four absorbent towel/fenestrated drape
- Chlorhexidine gluconate (ChloraPrep) or isopropyl alcohol for preoperative skin prep
- One 18–20 G × 3.5 inch Tuohy epidural needle or one 22 G 5-inch spinal needle
- Two 4 inch × 4 inch gauze dressings
- One 3 cc Luer lock syringes—contrast media
- One 5 cc Luer lock syringe—steroid cocktail

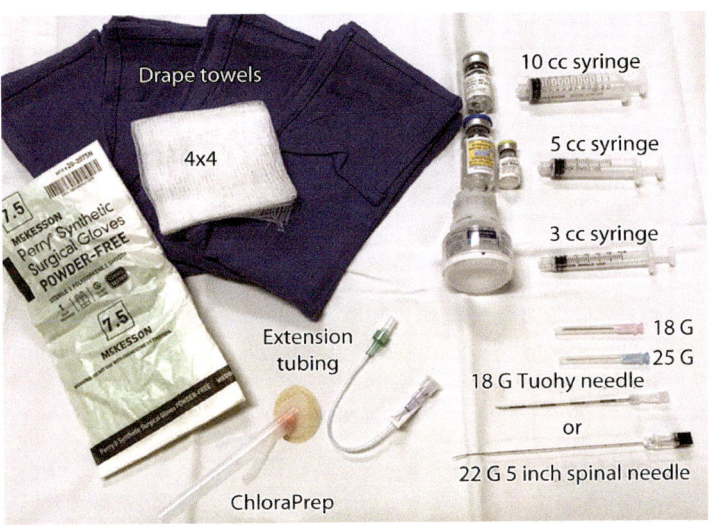

Fig. 1.3: Procedural kit.

- One 10 cc Luer lock syringe—local anesthetic transdermal infiltration
- One 10 mL LOR syringe with Luer slip tip [if an interlaminar epidural steroid injection (ESI) is performed]
- One 18 G × 1.5 inch needle—aspiration needle
- One 25 G × 1.5 inch needle—transdermal infiltration needle
- Extension tubing (minimizes needle movements and increases distance from radiation exposure)
- One set of 10 medication labels
- Band-aids.

The Needle (Fig. 1.4)
- Quincke type (cutting) needle
- *22 G 5-inch spinal needle*:
  ◊ May require less frequent adjustment compared to a 25 G
  ◊ 5 inch versus 3.5 inch:
     ◆ Do not find yourself short. A 5-inch needle can be used for about 90% of the blocks. Body habitus (BMI >30), oblique angulation, and block selection will determine the required length of the needle.
     ◆ Estimation of skin to the subarachnoid space depth (SSD) can be measured using Stocker's formula: SSD (mm) = $0.5 \times$ weight (kg) + 18^2
- *Distance taken from mid spinal level*:
  ◊ The needle moves in the direction of the bevel or *opposite to the notch*.
     ◆ Place a 5–10° bend away from the notch to improve steerability
     ◆ *Exception*: The Tuohy needle—the notch is on the same side as the curvature of the needle.

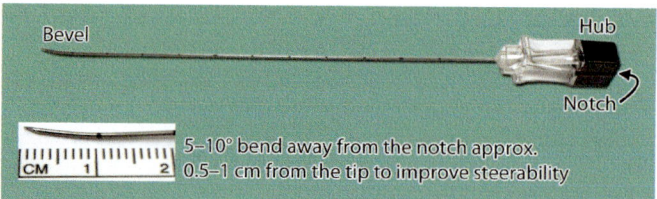

Fig. 1.4: Spinal needle.

- *Needle driving*:
    ◊ Needle driving skills come with experience. When first starting off, identify your target and place the C-arm laser aimer (if available) at the center of your target. Then, "light at the center of the hub!" Place the X-ray laser marker over the hub. This technique helps keep the needle aligned to the target producing a "gun barrel" view.

PAIN PROCEDURE CURRENT PROCEDURE TERMINOLOGY CODES (2017)[3]

> This list may not be all inclusive and is not intended to be used for coding/billing purposes. The final determination of reimbursement for services is the decision of the health plan and is based on the individual's policy or benefit entitlement structure as well as claims processing rules.

Craniofacial Blocks (Fluoroscopy is *not* Bundled)
- Trigeminal nerve (any branch): *64400*
- Sphenopalatine ganglion: *64505*

Sympathetic Blocks (Fluoroscopy is *not* Bundled)
- Stellate ganglion (cervical sympathetic): *64510*
- Superior hypogastric plexus: *64517*
- Thoracic or lumbar paravertebral sympathetic [lumbar sympathetic block (LSB)] or ganglion impar block: *64520*
- Celiac plexus: *64530*
- Splanchnic nerve block: *64530*

Peripheral Nerve Blocks (Fluoroscopy is *not* Bundled)
- Other peripheral nerve: *64450*
    ◊ Destruction: *64640*
- Pudendal nerve block: *64430*
- Intercostal nerve (single): *64420*
- Intercostal nerve (multiple): *64421*
- Coccygeal nerve block: *64450*

Interlaminar Epidural Steroid Injections (Fluoroscopy is Bundled)
- Interlaminar—cervical or thoracic: *62321*
- Interlaminar—lumbar or sacral (caudal): *62323*
- Epidural blood patch: *62273*

Transforaminal Epidural Steroid Injection (Fluoroscopy is Bundled)
- Transforaminal—cervical or thoracic (*first* level): *64479*
- Transforaminal—cervical or thoracic (*each additional* level): *64480*

Chapter 1: Basics to Fluoroscopy

- Transforaminal—lumbar or sacral (*first* level): *64483*
- Transforaminal—lumbar or sacral (*each additional* level): *64484*

Intra-articular Facet Joint or Medial Branch Block (Fluoroscopy is Bundled)
- Intra-articular joint or medial branch block (MBB)—cervical or thoracic (*first* level): *64490*
- Intra-articular joint or MBB—cervical or thoracic (*second* level): *64491*
- Intra-articular joint or MBB—cervical or thoracic (*third* level): *64492*
- Intra-articular joint or MBB—lumbar or sacral (*first* level): *64493*
- Intra-articular joint or MBB—lumbar or sacral (*second* level): *64494*
- Intra-articular joint or MBB—lumbar or sacral (*third* level): *64495*.

Note: Codes based upon spinal level/facet joint, not individual medial branches. Each facet joint is innervated by two different medial branch nerves. Hence, an L3-5 medial branch block, deinnervates the L4/5 and L5/S1 facet joint, therefore can only be billed as a first and second level procedure.

Facet Joint Radiofrequency Ablation (Fluoroscopy is *not* Bundled)
- Medial branch cervical or thoracic (*first* joint): *64633*
- Medial branch cervical or thoracic (*each additional* joint): *64634*
- Medial branch lumbar or sacral (*first* joint): *64635*
- Radiofrequency ablation (RFA)—lumbar or sacral (*each additional* joint): *64636*.

Spinal Cord Stimulator Trial—Cervical or Thoracolumbar (Fluoroscopy is Bundled)
- Percutaneous lead placement: *63650*—bill × 2 if trial required 2 leads
  ◊ Includes 10-day global period.

Discogram/Discography (Fluoroscopy is Bundled)
- Lumbar discogram/discography (each disk): *62290*.

Intrathecal Trial (Fluoroscopy is *not* Bundled)
- Injection of diagnostic substance (anesthetics, antispasmotics, opioids solutions) into the epidural or subarachnoid space: *62322*.

Joints and Bursa—Injection or Aspiration (Fluoroscopy is *not* Bundled)
- Major joint/bursa: *20610* (knee, hip, shoulder, trochanteric bursa, subacromial bursa, pes anserine bursa)
- Intermediate joint/bursa: *20605* (temporomandibular, acromioclavicular, wrist, elbow, ankle, olecranon bursa)
- Minor joint/bursa: *20600* [fingers proximal interphalangeal (PIP), distal interphalangeal (DIP), toes, carpometacarpal 20604]
- Sacroiliac joint (SIJ) with fluoroscopy: *27096*
- Sacral (S1-S3) lateral branch blocks: *64450* × 3
  ◊ Use 77003 instead of 77002
  ◊ RFA of L5 dorsal primary ramus and S1-S3 lateral branches: *64640* × 4
- Genicular nerve (knee) blocks: *64450* × 3 units
- Genicular nerve RFA: *64640* × 3.

Fluoroscopic Guidance (for Non-bundled Procedures)
- Fluoroscopic guidance for non-spinal procedures: *77002*
- Fluoroscopic guidance for spinal procedures: *77003*.

Modifiers
- Applies only to an office visit with a procedure: *25*
- Bilateral procedures: *50*
- Incomplete procedure (patient did not tolerate procedure): *52*
- Aborted procedure (patient's well-being at risk, i.e. vasovagal): *53*
- Distinct procedural service: *59*
  ◊ It is used on claims to indicate that two procedures reported during the same encounter are separate and distinct from each other and eligible for separate and unreduced payment.

TARGET ANGLES
Target angles have been described in Table 1.1.

Table 1.1: Description of target angles.

Procedure	Angles (based upon the C-arm intensifier)
Gasserian block	- Caudal tilt: 30–40° - Ipsilateral rotation: 15–20°
Mandibular and maxillary nerve block	- Lateral view
Sphenopalatine ganglion block	- Lateral view
Glossopharyngeal nerve block	- Lateral view
Cervical facet joint injection	- Caudal tilt: 25–35°
Atlantoaxial intra-articular injection	- AP view (optional—caudal tilt: 5–10°)
Cervical medial branch/TON/RFA	- Caudal tilt: 25–30° - Ipsilateral oblique versus 5–10°
Cervical ESI	- Caudal tilt: 5–15° - Contralateral oblique 45–55° (52)—for needle advancement and confirmation
Cervical transforaminal ESI	- Foraminal view: 40–50° (45)
Cervical spinal cord stimulation	- See cervical ESI with access at T1/2 interspace
Stellate ganglion	- C6; ipsilateral oblique 40–50° (45)
Glenohumeral joint injection	- AP view
Temporomandibular joint injection	- Lateral view
Thoracic facet joint injection	- AP view - Contralateral oblique (45–50°) for needle advancement
Thoracic medial branch/RFA	- AP view - Optional: Caudal tilt 5–10°, contralateral oblique 5–10°
Thoracic ESI	- Caudal tilt: 25–35°
Intercostal nerve block	- AP view - Optional: Caudal tilt 15–20°
Splanchnic	- Anterolateral margin of the T11 or T12 vertebral body - Ipsilateral oblique 5–10°

Contd....

Contd....

Procedure	Angles (based upon the C-arm intensifier)
Celiac plexus (transcrural technique)	▪ Target: Anterolateral margin of the L1 vertebral body ▪ Ipsilateral oblique 20–30° (TP aligns to the VB)
Superior hypogastric plexus block	▪ Target: Anterolateral margin of the L5 vertebral body ▪ Cephalad tilt: 20–30° ▪ Ipsilateral oblique: 25–35°
Ganglion impar/bilateral S5 and coccygeal nerve block	▪ AP view to confirm midline ▪ Lateral view for needle advancement
Pudendal nerve block	▪ Target: Ischial spine ▪ Caudal tilt: 5–10° ▪ Ipsilateral oblique: 5–10°
Lumbar ESI	▪ Caudal tilt: 5–15°
Subpedicular TFESI	▪ AP view (optional: ipsilateral oblique 5–10°)
Supraneural TFESI	▪ Ipsilateral oblique: 15–20°
Retroneural TFESI	▪ AP view (optional: ipsilateral oblique 5–10° until the lamina bisects the pedicle)
Infraneural TFESI	▪ Ipsilateral rotation: 30–35°
Caudal ESI	▪ AP view to determine midline ▪ Lateral view for needle advancement
Lumbar facet joint injection	▪ Ipsilateral oblique: 25–35°

Lumbar medial branch block (MBB)/RFA	▪ L1-4 MBB:
	  ♦ Ipsilateral oblique: 15–20°
	  ♦ Caudal/cephalad tilt:15–20°
	▪ L1-4 MBRFA:
	  ♦ Ipsilateral oblique: 15–20°
	  ♦ Caudal tilt:15–20°
	▪ L5 DRB/RFA:
	  ♦ Ipsilateral oblique: 0–5°
	  ♦ Caudal tilt: 0–5°

Lumbar discography	▪ Ipsilateral oblique 35–45° (SAP bisects the VB)
SCS-lumbar	▪ AP view ▪ Needle entry lateral to the pedicle below the target interspace at a 20–30° angle toward midline
Intrathecal trial	▪ Below the L1-2 interspace ▪ AP view
Sacroiliac joint injection	▪ Target: posterior, inferior SIJ opening ▪ Cephalad tilt: 10–15° ▪ Ipsilateral oblique: 5–10°
Sacral lateral branch block/RFA	▪ AP view (optional: Caudal tilt 0–5°; ipsilateral oblique 0–5°)
Lumbar sympathetic block	▪ Target inferior anterolateral margin of L2, or the anterolateral margins of L3, or L4 ▪ Ipsilateral oblique: 25–35°
Hip intra-articular injection	▪ AP view
Articular branches of the hip—femoral and obturator nerves	▪ Target: AIIS and the incisura of the acetabulum ▪ Caudal tilt: 10–15° ▪ Ipsilateral rotation: 0–5°
Knee intra-articular injection	▪ AP view
Genicular nerve block	▪ AP view

(RFA: Radiofrequency ablation; TON: Third occipital nerve; ESI: Epidural steroid injection; AP: Anteroposterior; TFESI: Transforaminal epidural steroid injection; SCS: Spinal cord stimulator; AIIS: Anterior Inferior Iliac Spine).

REFERENCES

1. Schueler BA. The AAPM/RSNA physics tutorial for residents: general overview of fluoroscopic imaging. Radiographics. 2000;20(4):1115-26.
2. Stocker DM, Bonsu B. A rule based on body weight for predicting the optimum depth of spinal needle insertion for lumbar puncture in children. Acad Emerg Med. 2005;5:105-6.
3. http://www.cms.gov/ICD10; accessed September 2017.

Chapter 2

Pharmacology

ANTICOAGULATION GUIDELINES

Anticoagulation guidelines have been described in Table 2.1.
- Table 2.1 is based upon the evidence-based guidelines published by the American Society of Regional Anesthesia and Pain Medicine, Third edition.

Table 2.1: Anticoagulation guidelines for interventional pain procedures

Drug	Stopping medication before intermediate to high-risk procedure	Restarting medication after procedure
Aspirin	Consider 6 days for high-risk procedure	24 hours
Apixaban (Eliquis)	3–5 days	24 hours
Clopidogrel (Plavix)	7 days	12–24 hours
Dabigatran (Pradaxa, Pradax, Prazaxa)	4–5 days 6 days if renal function impaired	24 hours
Enoxaparin (Lovenox) – Prophylaxis	12 hours	12–24 hours
Enoxaparin (Lovenox) – Therapeutic dose (1 mg/kg q12h or 1.5 mg/kg q day)	24 hours	12–24 hours
Heparin – IV vascular surgery	4 hours	2 hours 24 hours if was bloody
Heparin – SQ BID/TID prophylaxis	8–10 hours	2 hours
NSAIDs	5 half-lives	24 hours
Prasugrel (Efficient)	7–10 days	12–24 hours
Rivaroxaban (Xarelto)	3 days	24 hours
Ticagrelor (Brilinta, Brilique, Possia)	5 days	12–24 hours
Warfarin (Coumadin)	5 days AND normal INR	24 hours

(SQ: Subcutaneously; NSAIDs: Nonsteroidal anti-inflammatory drugs).
- The table is based upon the evidence-based multi-society guidelines ("Interventional Spine and Pain Procedures in Patients on Antiplatelet and Anticoagulant Medications: Guidelines From the American Society of Regional Anesthesia and Pain Medicine, the European Society of Regional Anesthesia and Pain Therapy, the American Academy of Pain Medicine, the International Neuromodulation Society, the North American Neuromodulation Society, and the World Institute of Pain," Regional Anesthesia & Pain Medicine: May/June 2015 - Volume 40 - Issue 3 - p 182–212)
- No recommendations were given regarding superficial nerve blocks in patients receiving superficial peripheral nerve blocks
- If an indwelling catheter is to be placed, refer to these guidelines for further guidance on how to plan medication dosing around placement and removal of a catheter.

- No recommendations were given regarding superficial nerve blocks in patients receiving superficial peripheral nerve blocks.
- If an indwelling catheter is to be placed, refer to these guidelines for further guidance on how to plan medication dosing around placement and removal of a catheter.

LOCAL ANESTHETICS

Mechanism of Action

- Two different classes: (1) ester and (2) amides.
- Blockade of voltage-gated sodium channels.

Pharmacodynamics/Pharmacokinetics[1]

Local anesthetic pharmacology have been described in Table 2.2.
- Clinically, the order of loss of nerve function is a followed: (1) pain, (2) temperature, (3) touch, (4) proprioception, and (5) skeletal muscle tone.
- *Onset*: Determined by tissue pH, the pKa of the local anesthetic, and the amount of non-ionized drug available.
- *Duration*: Action depends on plasma and protein binding.
- *Potency*: It is related to lipid solubility.
- The uptake of local anesthetic from greatest to least as is follows: IV > tracheal > intercostal > caudal > paracervical > epidural > brachial plexus > sciatic > subcutaneous.
- Amino-amide local anesthetics are cleared form plasma by hepatic metabolism, primarily via oxidative dealkylation.
- Ester local anesthetics are metabolized by pseudocholinesterase and partially by red blood cell esterases.

Local Anesthetic Complications

- *Allergy to local anesthetics*:
  ◊ Ester local anesthetics are metabolized to para-aminobenzoic acid (PABA), a known allergen.
  ◊ Methylparaben, a preservative in both ester and amide local anesthetic solutions, is also metabolized to PABA
- *Central nervous system (CNS) toxicity*: Perioral numbness, metallic taste, light-headedness, visual and auditory disturbances, dizziness, paresthesia, unconsciousness, convulsions, coma, and respiratory depression.[2]

Table 2.2: Local anesthetic pharmacology.[4]

Agent	Onset	Equipotency anesthetic concentration	Approximate anesthetic duration (min)	Recommended maximum single dose (mg/kg)
Lidocaine (Xylocaine)	Intermediate	1	60–120	4 (7 with epi)
Mepivacaine (Carbocaine)	Intermediate	1	90–180	4 (7 with epi)
Ropivacaine (Naropin)	Slow	0.5	180–480	3
Bupivacaine (Marcaine)	Slow	0.25	180–480	3

(Epi: Epinephrine)

- *Cardiovascular toxicity*: Hypotension, tachycardia, electrocardiography abnormalities (prolonged PR interval and QRS), and cardiac arrest.[2]
- *Intralipid 20% fat emulsion*:
  ◊ Recommended dosage: 1.5 mL/kg bolus (repeated up to a total of 5 mL/kg), followed by infusion of 10 mL/min.[3]

STEROIDS

Mechanism of Action

Inhibiting prostaglandin synthesis, impairs the cell-mediated and humoral immune responses, and block nociceptive C fiber conduction.

Selection of Glucocorticoids

- Recommendations are based upon clinical experience and personal preference.
- Intra-articular injections—triamcinolone is more effective in pain reduction than other corticosteroids.[3]
- Transforaminal injections, head and neck and any other procedure where there is a high risk for an intravascular injection—use non-particulate steroids, i.e. dexamethasone and betamethasone
  ◊ There is one questionable case report that documents adverse CNS effects from non-particulates during a transforaminal injection versus a complication resulting from vascular penetration, i.e. vasospasm, thrombus formation or a dissection[6]
  ◊ Studies demonstrate no significant differences in pain reduction or the number of repeat injections with particulate compared with non-particulate transforaminal epidural steroid injection.[7]

Frequency of Injections

- Insufficient evidence to determine how many steroid injections one can receive in a year.
- North American Spine Society determined that for transforaminal epidural steroid injections (TFESIs):[8]
  ◊ No more than two injections to achieve a beneficial response
  ◊ Up to three injections in a 6-month period to reinstate and maintain benefit
    ◆ Benefit—reduced pain and/or improved function, along with reduced need for other health care.
- More than four injections per year—an alternative treatment should be considered (i.e. surgical consult, changes in medication management).

Maximum Dose

- Previous research suggests triamcinolone dosage more than or equal to 3 mg/kg/year (administration route unspecified), or the equivalent, should be limited to prevent corticosteroid-induced bone loss.[9]
- Recent research suggests bone loss does not occur until the dose of triamcinolone, administered in the epidural space, is around 400 mg/year.

Side Effects

- Alterations in skin pigmentation (avoid tracking of steroids when withdrawing the needle).
- Tendon rupture, cartilage damage, pericapsular calcification and bone mineral loss are all potential side effects that can worsen patient outcomes.[10]
- All long-acting glucocorticoids, with the exception of dexamethasone, contain preservatives. Intrathecal administration carries an increased risk for arachnoiditis.
- Patients with hemoglobin A1c levels greater than or equal to 7% have elevations in blood glucose that are higher and last longer (4–5 days) than patients with lower levels. There is no established "safe" cut off value for blood glucose levels prior to epidural administration of corticosteroids but, most practitioners utilize a cut off around 200 mg/dL.

Commercially Available Steroid Preparations

Commercially available steroid preparations have been given in Table 2.3.

CONTRAST AGENTS

- Iodine based radiopaque agent: Ionic:
  - High-osmolarity contrast media (HOCM):
    - Causes severe irritation and more likely to cause vasodilatation, increased capillary permeability, and mast cell degranulation
    - Hence more likely to cause an allergic reaction
  - Not commonly used in pain practices
- Nonionic—iohexol (Omnipaque) and iopamidol (Isovue)
  - Low-osmolarity contrast media (LOCM)—although still hyperosmolar compare to serum
  - Dose based upon the iodine concentration, standard dose for pain procedures— between 200 mg and 300 mg/dL
  - Omnipaque can be used for intrathecal use, Isovue is not Food and Drug Administration (FDA) approved
  - Four- to fivefold reduction in all reactions compared to HOCM.

Table 2.3: Commercially available steroid preparations.

Drug	IM dose (mg)	Approximate equivalent dose	Relative glucocorticoids (anti-inflammatory)	Relative mineralocorticoid (Na retention)	Half-life (hours)
Triamcinolone acetonide (Kenalog)	40–80	4	5	0	12–36
Betamethasone (Celestone)	9	0.6	25	0	36–72
Methylprednisolone (Depomedrol)	40–80	4	5	0.5	18–36
Dexamethasone acetate (Decadron)	4–8	0.75	25	0	36–54

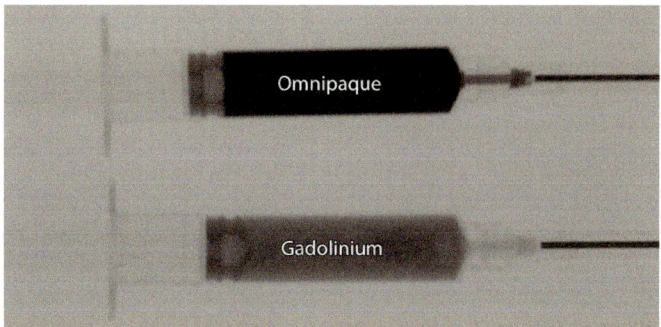

Fig. 2.1: Gadolinium produces a dispersal pattern that is less distinct than iodinated contrast media.

Gadolinium (OptiMARK) (Fig. 2.1)
- Alternative contrast media used for patients with a true history of an allergic reaction to nonionic contrast.
- Not FDA approved for intrathecal use.
- Not proven safer than the iodinated contrast agents and should be limited to 3 mL. Paramagnetic properties, hence also called MRI contrast.

Adverse Reactions
- Ninety percent of adverse reactions with nonionic contrast materials are anaphylactoid.
- *Mild reactions*: Localized hives, itching, rhinorrhea, mild nausea and vomiting, coughing, and lightheadedness.
- *Moderate reactions*: Generalized hives, mild bronchospasm, swelling, and hypotension.
- *Severe reactions*: Severe hypotension, severe bronchospasm, aseptic meningitis, arachnoiditis (seen in both iodinated contrast and gadolinium), seizures, and death.
- Medical myth-allergies to shellfish = allergies to iodine[11]
  - ◊ Patients are allergic to the protein in shellfish and not iodine.

REFERENCES
1. Horlocker TT. Local anesthetic agents: pharmacology. In: Murray MJ, Rose SH, Wedel DJ, Wass CT, Harrison BA, Mueller JT (Eds). Faust's Anesthesiology Review, 4th edition. Philadelphia: Elsevier Saunders; 2015. pp. 269-71.
2. Cusato M, Niebel T, Bettinelli S, et al. How pharmacokinetic can help to choose the right local anesthetics during epidural infusion. Eur J Pain Suppl. 2011;5(2):471-5.
3. Drasner K. Local anesthetics. In: Miller R, Pardo MG Jr (Eds). Basics of Anesthesia, 6th edition. Philadelphia: Elsevier Saunders; 2011. pp. 130-41.
4. Williams DJ, Walker JD. A nomogram for calculating the maximum dose of local anaesthetic. Anaesthesia. 2014;69:847-53.
5. Hepper CT, Halvorson JJ, Duncan ST, et al. The efficacy and duration of intra-articular corticosteroid injection for knee osteoarthritis: a systematic review of level I studies. J Am Acad Orthop Surg. 2009;17(10):638-46.
6. Gharibo C, Fakhry M, Diwan S, et al. Conus medullaris infarction after a right L4 transforaminal epidural steroid injection using dexamethasone. Pain Physician. 2016;19(8):E1211-4.

7. Kennedy DJ, Plastaras C, Casey E, et al. Comparative effectiveness of lumbar transforaminal epidural steroid injections with particulate versus nonparticulate corticosteroids for lumbar radicular pain due to intervertebral disc herniation: a prospective, randomized, double-blind trial. Pain Med. 2014;15:548-55.
8. North American Spine Society. Lumbar transforaminal epidural steroid injections review and recommendation statement. (2013). [online] Available at www.spine.org/Documents/ResearchClinicalCare/LTFESIREviewREcStatement.pdf [Accessed August 2017].
9. Kim N, Schroeder J, Hoffler CE, et al. Elevated hemoglobin A1C levels correlate with blood glucose elevation in diabetic patients following local corticosteroid injection in the hand: a prospective study. Plast Reconstr Surg. 2015;136(4):474e-9e.
10. Bouvard B, Legrand E, Audran M, et al. Glucocorticoid-induced osteoporosis: a review. Clin Rev Bone Miner Metab. 2010;8(1):15-26.
11. Schabelman E, Witting M. The relationship of radiocontrast, iodine, and seafood allergies: a medical myth exposed. J Emerg Med. 2010;39(5):701-7.

Chapter 3

Head, Neck and Upper Extremity

GASSERIAN GANGLION BLOCK (FIGS. 3.1 TO 3.5)

Indication
Treatment of facial pain (trigeminal neuralgia) in the trigeminal nerve distribution.

Advantage
Radiofrequency ablation (RFA) or chemoneurolysis can be performed for prolonged benefit.

Disadvantages/Complications
- High risk for intravascular injection, cerebrospinal fluid (CSF) aspiration, and total spinal block.
- Common side effects include worsening headache and nausea.

Injectate
4–8 mg of dexamethasone +1 mL of bupivacaine 0.75–0.5%.

Techniques
1. *Patient position*: Supine with slight neck extension.

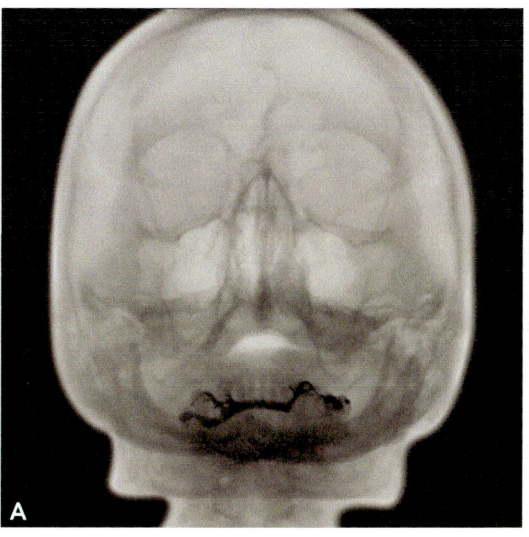 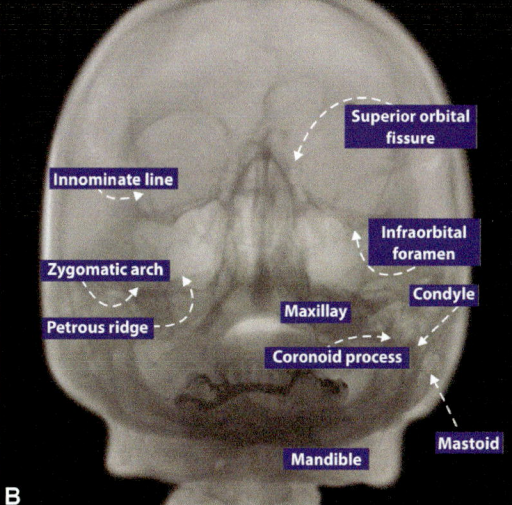

Figs. 3.1A and B: (A) Gasserian ganglion block—anteroposterior (AP) view; (B) Gasserian ganglion block: AP view (labeled). Gross overview of landmarks.

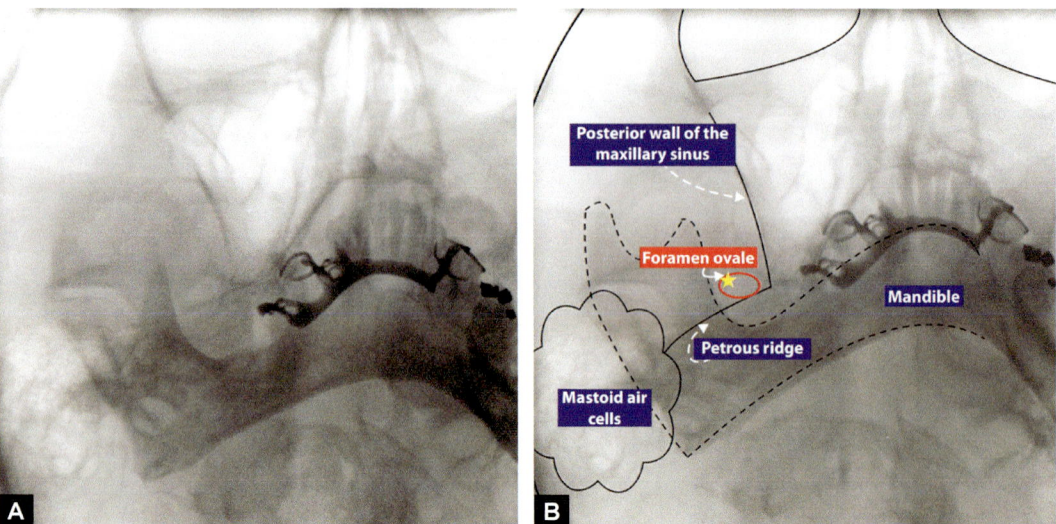

Figs. 3.2A and B: (A) Gasserian ganglion block: Initial starting angle (modified Water's view). Identify the posterior wall of the maxillary sinus, the petrous ridge, and the mastoid air cells. The foramen ovale lies superior to the petrous ridge about one-third of the distance between the posterior wall of the maxillary sinus and the mastoid air cells. (B) Gasserian ganglion block: starting angle (labeled).

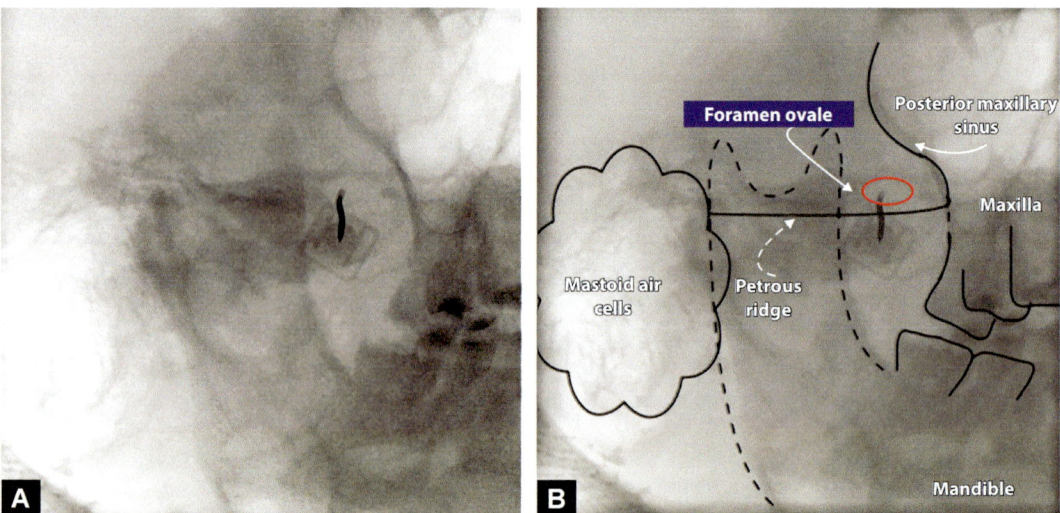

Figs. 3.3A and B: (A) Gasserian ganglion block: starting angle; (B) Gasserian ganglion block: starting angle (labeled).

2. *Target*: Through the foramen ovale, 3–5 mm superficial to the clivus (safe boundry).
3. *Optimize view*: Foramen ovale lies superior to the petrous ridge about one-third of the distance between the posterior wall of the maxillary sinus and the mastoid air cells. Therefore, tracing the maxillary molars can help identify the posterior edge of the maxilla and the maxillary sinus.

Chapter 3: Head, Neck and Upper Extremity

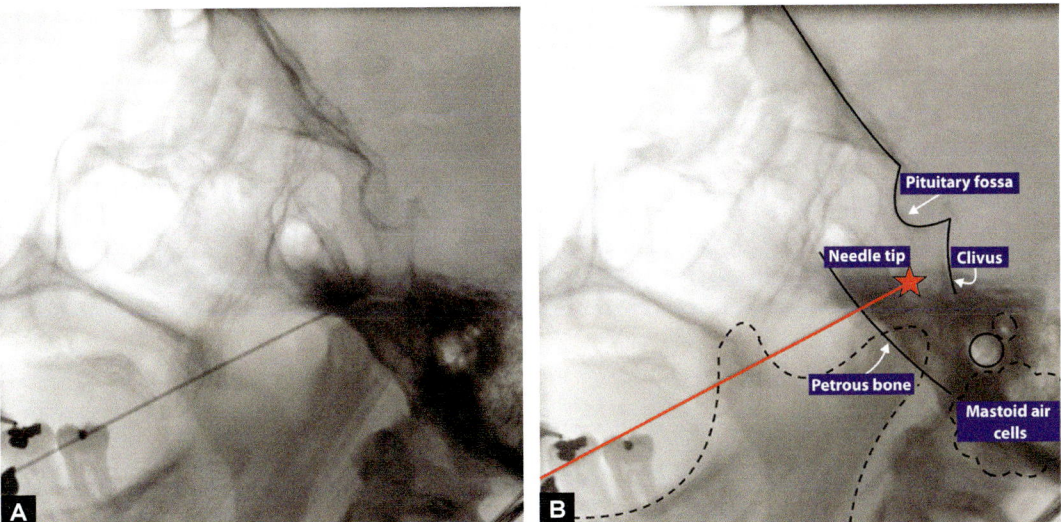

Figs. 3.4A and B: (A) Gasserian ganglion block—lateral view. Advance past the petrous bone (Latin for "stone/rock", hence it is darker than the surrounding structures). Accidental cerebrospinal fluid (CSF) aspiration may be encountered if the needle is advanced past the clivus. Pull back the needle until there is no return of CSF and do not inject local anesthetics; (B) Gasserian ganglion block—lateral view (labeled).

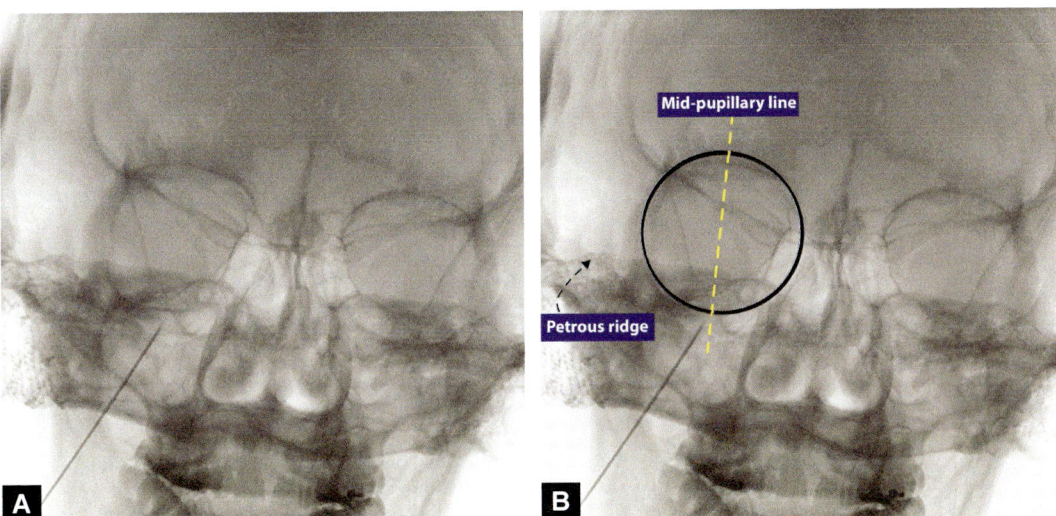

Figs. 3.5A and B: (A) Gasserian ganglion block anteroposterior (AP) view. Once past the petrous bone, confirm needle placement. The needle should lie at the mid-pupillary line; (B) Gasserian ganglion block—AP view (labeled).

- Start in anteroposterior (AP) view
- Then rotate ipsilateral 15–20°
- Then tilt caudal 30–40°.
4. Advance spinal needle (3.5 inch × 25 G) toward the superior or inferior edge of the foramen ovale. Check lateral view periodically to determine depth.

- Once the petrous bone is contacted, redirect the needle inferiorly or superiorly into the foramen.
- Once in the foramen, continue advancing in lateral view.
5. *Lateral view*: Advance needle toward, but not beyond, the clivus until it is at the target described above.
6. *Anteroposterior view*: Confirm that tip is at the mid-pupillary line.
7. Confirm placement with contrast under live fluoroscopy in both AP and lateral views.

MAXILLARY AND MANDIBULAR NERVE BLOCK (FIGS. 3.6A TO C)

Indication

Treatment of facial pain specifically in a selective nerve distribution (V2 and V3 divisions of the trigeminal nerve).

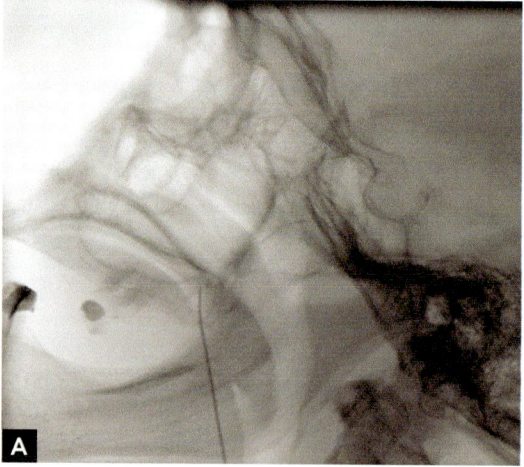

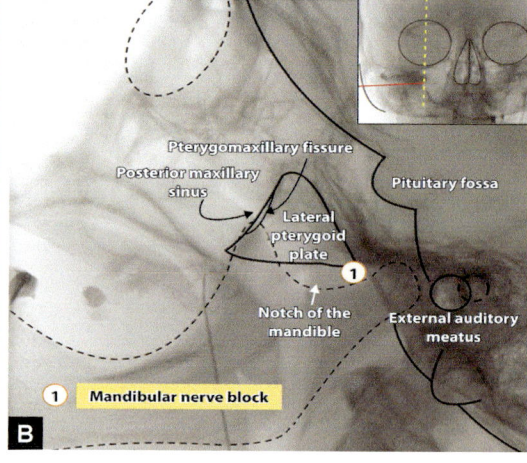

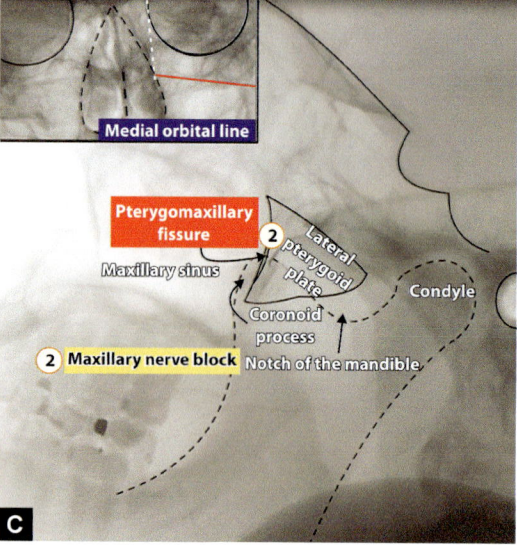

Figs. 3.6A to C: Maxillary and mandibular nerve block: Lateral view. Identify the lateral pterygoid plate which lies posterior to the maxillary sinus. The pterygomaxillary fissure connects to the pterygopalatine fossa which houses the maxillary nerve, superiorly, and the sphenopalatine ganglion (pterygopalatine ganglion), inferiorly. The mandibular nerve lies at the posterosuperior border of the lateral pterygoid plate. The posterosuperior border of the lateral pterygoid plate can be identified by drawing an imaginary vertical line anterior to pituitary fossa (sella turcica) and inferior to the petrous bone; (B) The mandibular nerve (V3) enters the infratemporal fossa via the foramen ovale. Confirmation of needle placement is in the anteroposterior (AP) view. The needle should lie at the mid-pupillary line—lateral view (labeled); (C) The maxillary nerve is the second branch of the trigeminal nerve (V2)—lateral view (labeled). It passes from the middle cranial fossa into the pterygopalatine fossa through the foramen rotundum. Confirmation of needle placement is in the AP view. The needle should lie lateral to the nasal mucosa near the medial orbital line.

Advantage
Radiofrequency ablation or chemoneurolysis can be performed for prolonged benefit.

Disadvantages/Complications
High risk for intravascular injection, CSF aspiration, hematoma, and a total spinal block.

Injectate
4–8 mg of dexamethasone + 1 mL of bupivacaine 0.25–0.5%.

Techniques
1. *Patient position*: Supine with neck in slight extension.
2. Target (relative to lateral pterygoid plate):
   - *Mandibular nerve*: 1–2 mm past posterosuperior border
   - *Maxillary nerve*: 1–2 mm past AP border toward the pterygomaxillary fissure.
3. *Lateral view*: Identify the lateral pterygoid plate:
   - Plate lies just posterior to the maxillary sinus
   - It is visible through the mandibular notch between the coronoid and condylar processes.
4. Advance a spinal needle (3.5 inch × 22–25 G) toward the respective border of the pterygoid plate (i.e. posterosuperior border for mandibular nerve block).
5. Once contact is made with the lateral pterygoid plate, walk off 1–2 mm.
6. *Anteroposterior view*: Tip should lie at the edge of the medial orbital line.
7. Confirm placement with contrast under live fluoroscopy.

SPHENOPALATINE GANGLION BLOCK (FIGS. 3.7 AND 3.8)
Indication
Treatment of atypical facial, headaches [including post-dural puncture headache (PDPH)], pain in the maxillary teeth or gums, and chronic regional pain syndrome (CRPS) of the face.

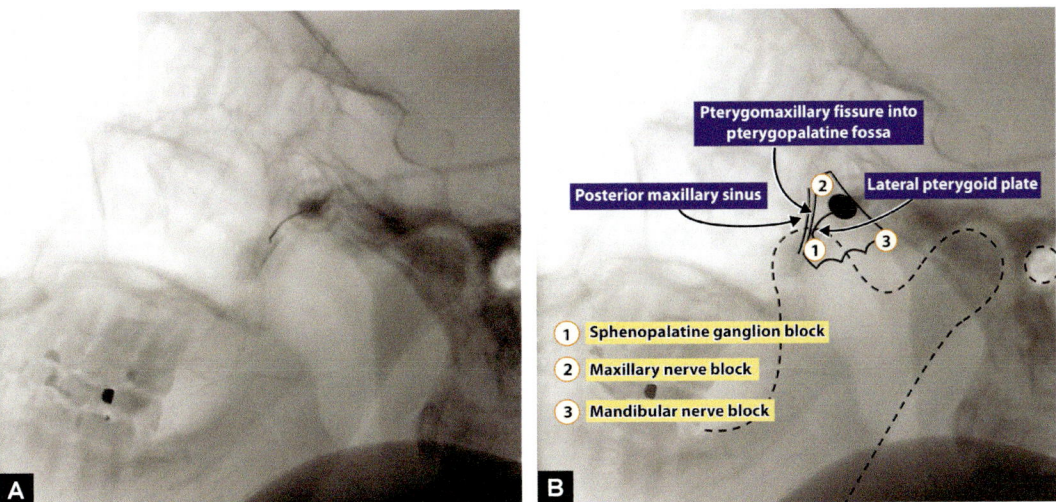

Figs. 3.7A and B: (A) Sphenopalatine ganglion block—lateral view. The sphenopalatine is a parasympathetic ganglion found in the pterygopalatine fossa; (B) Sphenopalatine ganglion block—lateral view.

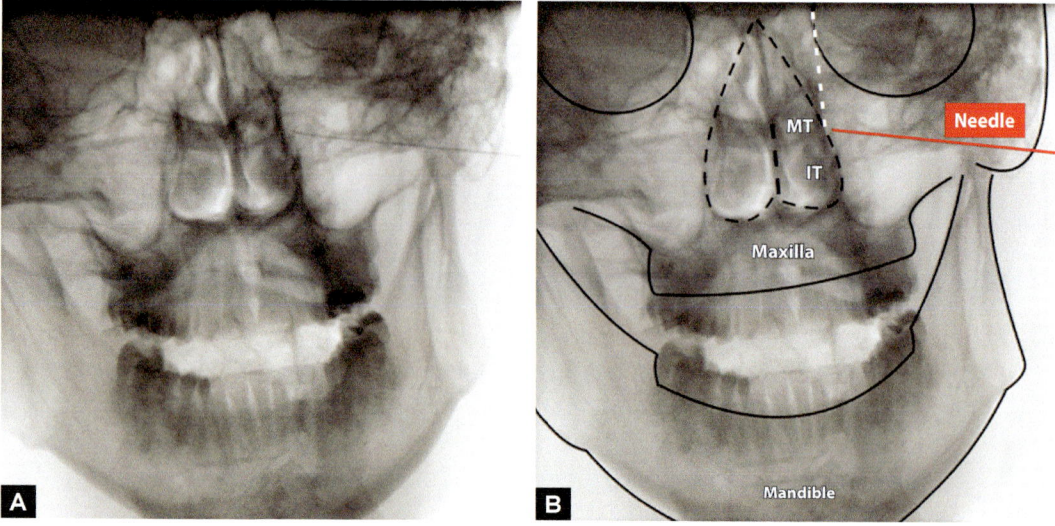

Figs. 3.8A and B: (A) Sphenopalatine ganglion block—anteroposterior (AP) view. Confirmation of needle placement. Needle placed at the superior-lateral margin of the nasal mucosa (lateral to the middle turbinate); (B) Sphenopalatine ganglion block—AP view (labeled).
(MT: Middle turbinate; IT: Inferior turbinate).

Advantage
Radiofrequency ablation or chemoneurolysis can be performed for prolonged benefit.

Disadvantages/Complications
High risk for intravascular injection, CSF aspiration, hematoma, and a total spinal block.

Injectate
4–8 mg of dexamethasone + 1 mL of bupivacaine 0.25–0.5%.

Techniques
1. *Patient position:* Supine with neck in slight extension.
2. *Target:* 1–2 mm past the anteroinferior border of the lateral pterygoid plate.
3. *Lateral view:* Identify the lateral pterygoid plate and the pterygomaxillary fissure.
    - Plate lies just posterior to the maxillary sinus
    - It is visible through the mandibular notch between the coronoid and condylar processes.
4. Advance a spinal needle (3.5 inch × 22–25 G) toward the anterior border of the plate.
5. Once contact is made with the lateral pterygoid plate, walk off anteriorly and inferiorly 1–2 mm.
6. *Anteroposterior view:* Tip should lie at the edge of the medial orbital line and lateral to the nasal mucosa
7. Confirm placement with contrast under live fluoroscopy.

GLOSSOPHARYNGEAL NERVE BLOCK (FIGS. 3.9 AND 3.10)
Indications
- Glossopharyngeal neuralgia (pain with swallowing, chewing, talking, foreign body sensation in throat, and atypical symptoms include tinnitus)

Chapter 3: Head, Neck and Upper Extremity   21

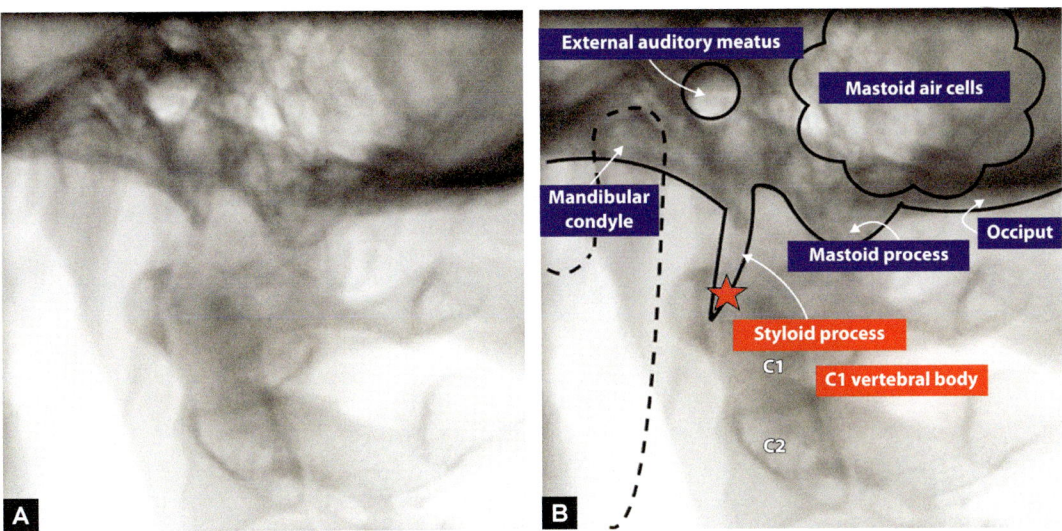

Figs. 3.9A and B: (A) Glossopharyngeal nerve block—lateral view. Identify the styloid process. The styloid process lies directly inferior to the external auditory meatus; (B) Glossopharyngeal nerve block—lateral view (labeled).

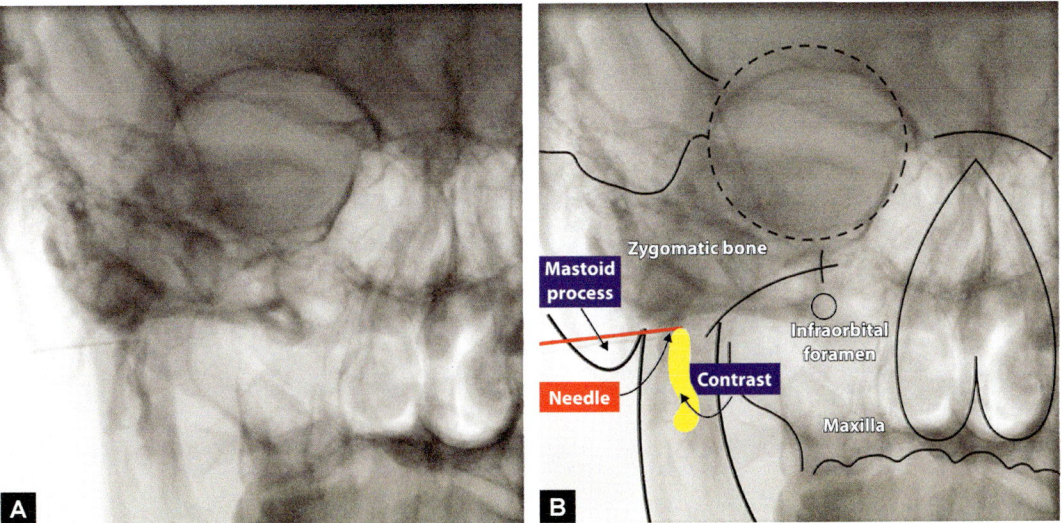

Figs. 3.10A and B: (A) Glossopharyngeal nerve block—anteroposterior (AP) view. Confirmation of needle placement. The styloid process should be met at a depth of 2–3 cm; (B) Glossopharyngeal nerve block—AP view (labeled).

- Eagle's syndrome
- Cancer related pain in the throat, tonsils, and posterior tongue.

Advantages
- Diagnostic and therapeutic block
- If successful, can proceed to pulsed RFA for prolonged benefit.

Disadvantages/Complications

High risk for intravascular injection (carotid and the internal jugular are located just medial to the glossopharyngeal nerve), hematoma, dysphagia, vagus nerve block. Bilateral injections should never be performed.

Injectate

4–8 mg of dexamethasone + 1 mL of bupivacaine 0.25–0.5%.

Techniques

1. *Patient position*: Supine
2. *Target*: Half-way between the angle of the mandible and mastoid process approximately 1–2 mm posteroinferiorly past the styloid process.
3. *Lateral view*: Identify angle of the mandible and the mastoid process.
   - Styloid process lies at the midpoint between the two structures.
   - Lies directly inferior to the external auditory meatus.
4. Advance spinal needle (3.5 inch × 22–25 G) toward the inferior aspect of the styloid process.
5. Contact the styloid process and walk off posteroinferiorly 1–2 mm.
6. Confirm placement with contrast in both AP and lateral views.

CERVICAL FACET INTRA-ARTICULAR INJECTION (FIGS. 3.11 TO 3.13)

Indications

- Cervical spondylosis
- Axial neck pain without radicular symptoms
- Occipital or cervicogenic headaches.

Advantages

Intra-articular injections are diagnostic and therapeutic interventions.

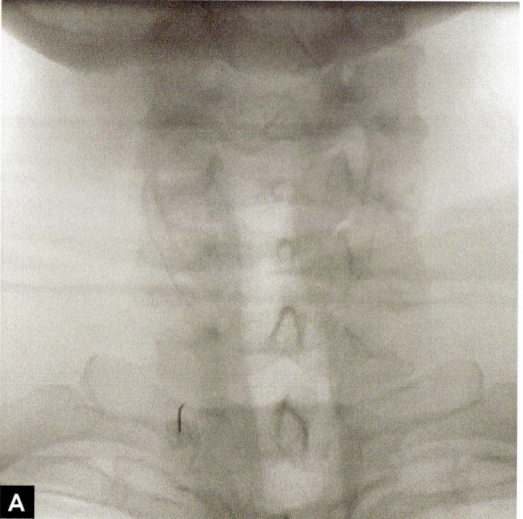 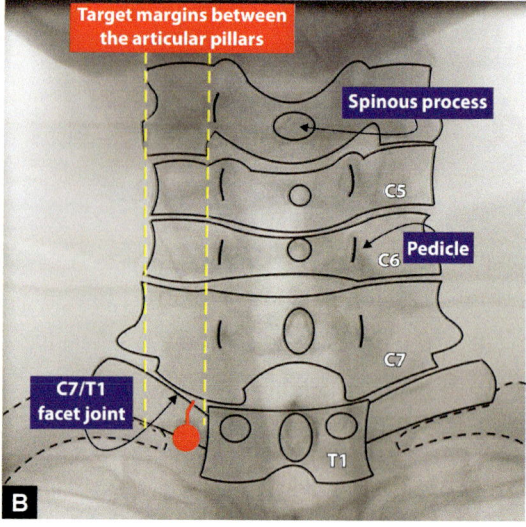

Figs. 3.11A and B: (A) Cervical intra-articular facet injection—caudal tilt 25–35°. Target the midpoint of the articular pillars; (B) Cervical intra-articular facet injection—caudal tilt 25–35° (labeled).

Chapter 3: Head, Neck and Upper Extremity

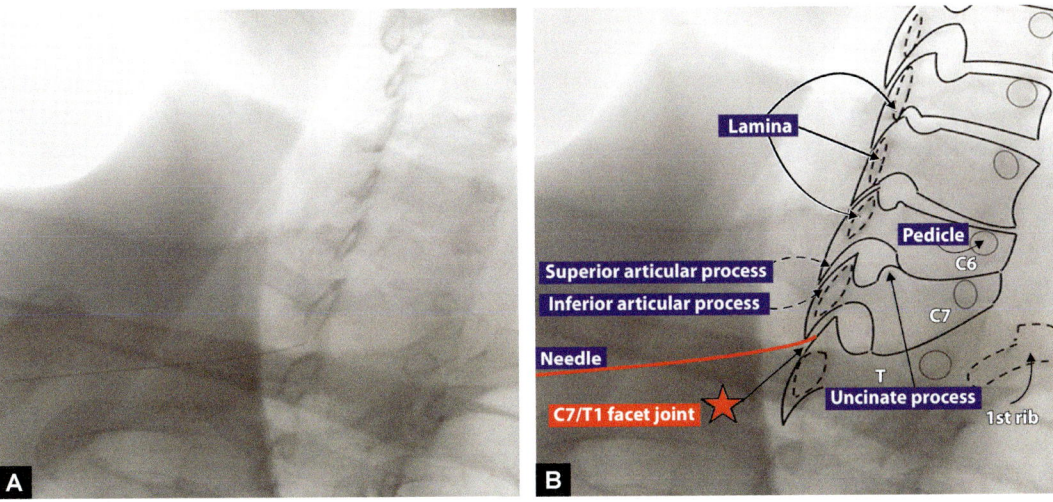

Figs. 3.12A and B: (A) Cervical facet intra-articular injection—contralateral oblique view (50–55°). Confirm needle placement via a lateral or contralateral oblique view; (B) Cervical facet intra-articular injection—contralateral oblique view (50–55°) (labeled).

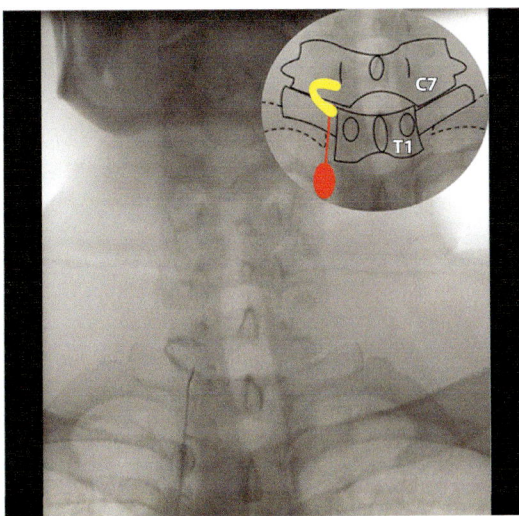

Fig. 3.13: Cervical facet intra-articular injection—anteroposterior (AP) view. The contrast spread should appear to be an elliptical shape. A maximum volume of 1 mL of the mixture of steroid and local anesthetics may be injection. An increase volume may result in the injectate flowing into an extradural space dorsal to the ligamentum flavum called "the retrodural space of Okada".[1,2]

Disadvantage/Complication
Worsening pain, epidural spread if volume of injectate is more than 1.5 mL.

Injectate
0.5–1 mL of 40–80 mg of methylprednisolone or steroid of choice + bupivacaine 0.5% divided among the joints.

Techniques
1. *Patient position*: Prone with small pillow under forehead or head rest apparatus.
2. *Target*: Intra-articular location approximately midpoint of the articular pillars.

3. *Anteroposterior view*: Tilt caudally 25–35° to improve visualization of joint.
4. Advance spinal needle (3.5 inch × 22–25 G) toward the joint line. Contact lamina.
5. *Contralateral oblique view*: Advance in this view until tip rests in the joint. A lateral view can also used for needle advancement
6. Confirm placement with a small amount of contrast (0.2–0.3 cc)

ATLANTOAXIAL INTRA-ARTICULAR INJECTION (FIGS. 3.14 AND 3.15)

Indications
- Cervical spondylosis
- Upper neck pain without radicular symptoms exacerbated by lateral rotation
- Occipital or cervicogenic headaches.

Advantage
Intra-articular injections are diagnostic and therapeutic interventions.

Disadvantages/Complications
- High risk for a neurovascular injection due to proximity of vertebral artery (just lateral to facet).
- Risk of spinal cord injury (medial to facet).
- C2 paresthesia
- Because of the risks involved, consider a third occipital nerve (TON) block prior to this procedure.

Injectate
0.5–1 mL of a 1:1 mixture of 40 mg of methylprednisolone or steroid of choice + bupivacaine 0.5%.

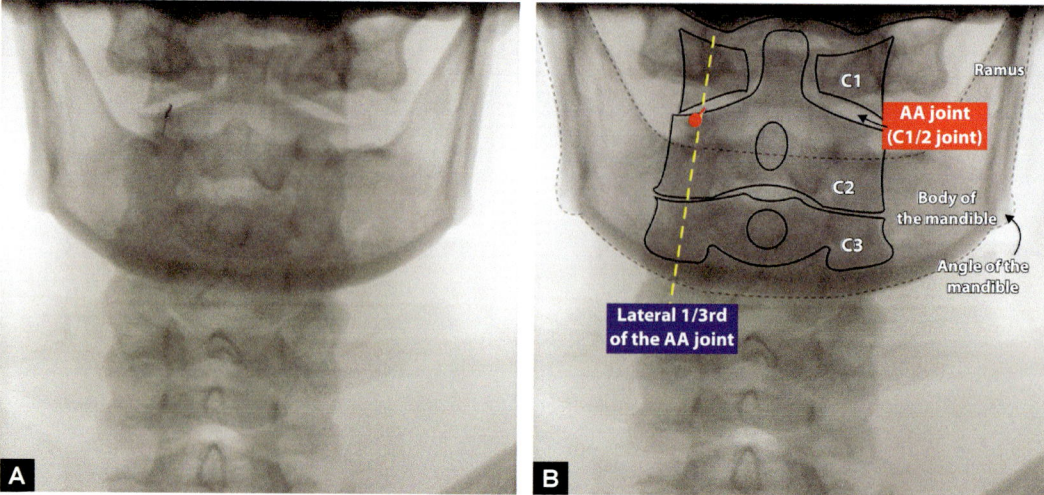

Figs. 3.14A and B: (A) Atlantoaxial intra-articular injection—anteroposterior (AP) view. Target the lateral one-third of the joint to avoid the vertebral artery (lateral to the facet joint), and the spinal cord (medial to the facet joint); (B) Atlantoaxial intra-articular injection—AP view (labeled).
(AA: Atlantoaxial).

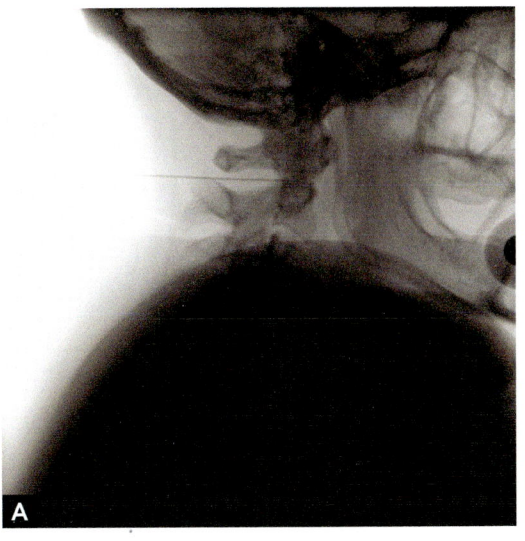 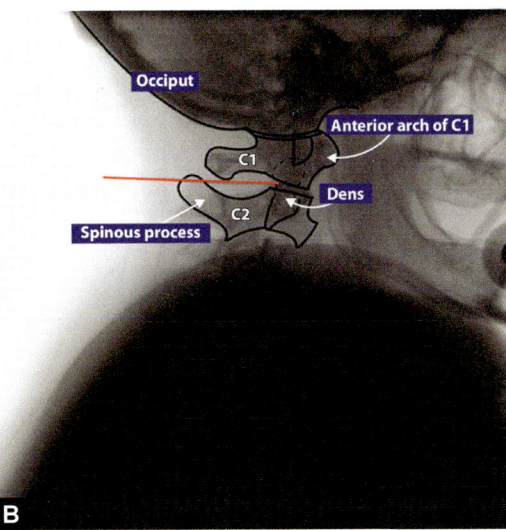

Figs. 3.15A and B: (A) Atlantoaxial intra-articular injection—lateral view. Needle placed at the posterior joint margin; (B) Atlantoaxial intra-articular injection—lateral view (labeled).

Techniques
1. *Patient position*: Prone with small pillow under forehead or head rest apparatus.
2. *Target*: Junction point of the lateral one-third and medial 2/3rd of the C1-2 joint.
3. *AP view*: Identify the posterior arch of the atlas (portion that encircles the dens):
   - Tilt caudally so that the arch is not obscuring the C1-2 joint (approximate 5–10°)
   - May need to ask patient to open mouth or rotate ipsilateral less than 5° to clear oral structures from obscuring joint.
4. Advance spinal needle (3.5 inch × 22–25 G) toward the target.
5. Contact the edge of C2 superior articular process (SAP).
6. *Lateral view*: Advance in this view until tip rests within joint (approximately 2–3 mm)
7. Confirm placement with a small amount of contrast under live fluoroscopy in both AP and lateral views.

CERVICAL MEDIAL BRANCH BLOCKS AND RADIOFREQUENCY ABLATION (FIGS. 3.16 TO 3.18)

Indications
- Cervical spondylosis/facet arthrosis
- Axial neck pain without radicular symptoms
- Occipital or cervicogenic headaches.

Advantages
- Medial branch block (MBB) provides diagnostic information.
- Chemoneurolytic ablation can be easily done using the MBB technique and by administering a chemoneurolytic substance (phenol, methylene blue, 50% dextrose).
- Radiofrequency ablation provides longer lasting relief.

Disadvantages/Complications
- Diagnostic blocks provide short-term duration (<12 hours if only bupivacaine is used).
- Minimal sedatives can falsify diagnostic information (i.e. giving midazolam causes muscle relaxation, and fentanyl can diminish pain scores).
- Requires multiple levels of injections as each joint is innervated by the two medial branches at the level (i.e. C4-C5 joint by C4 MB and C5 MB).

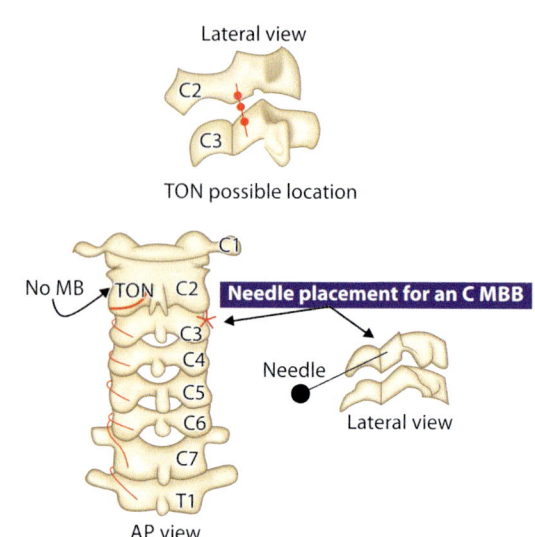

Fig. 3.16: Illustration of the cervical medial branches and location of needle placement. (MBB: Medial branch block; TON: Third occipital nerve; AP: Anteroposterior).

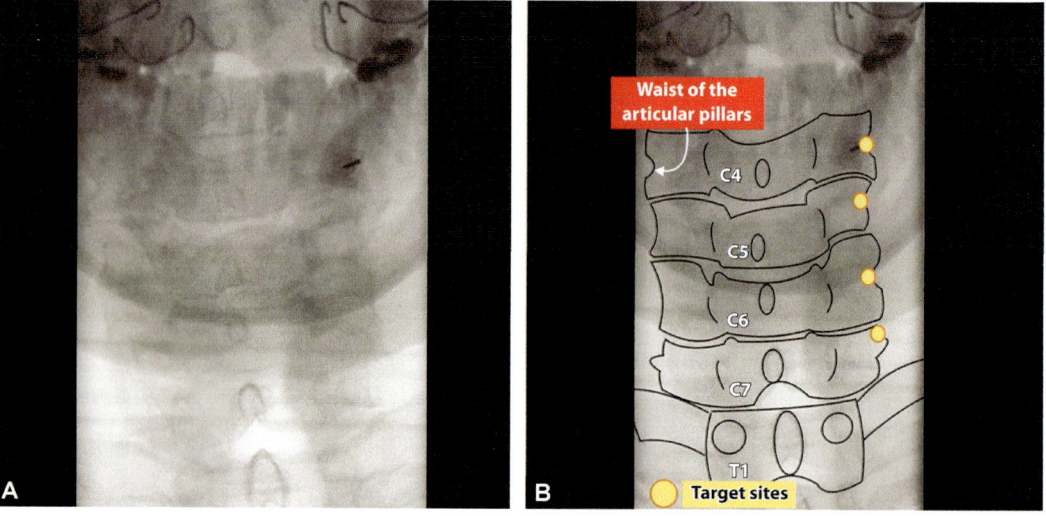

Figs. 3.17A and B: Cervical medial branch block/radiofrequency ablation (RFA)—anteroposterior (AP) view. Target the waist of the articular pillars. To improve visualization tilt caudal 20–30° and rotate ipsilateral 10–20°; (B) Cervical medial branch block/RFA—caudal tilt 20–30° and an ipsilateral rotation of 5–10° (labeled).

Chapter 3: Head, Neck and Upper Extremity 27

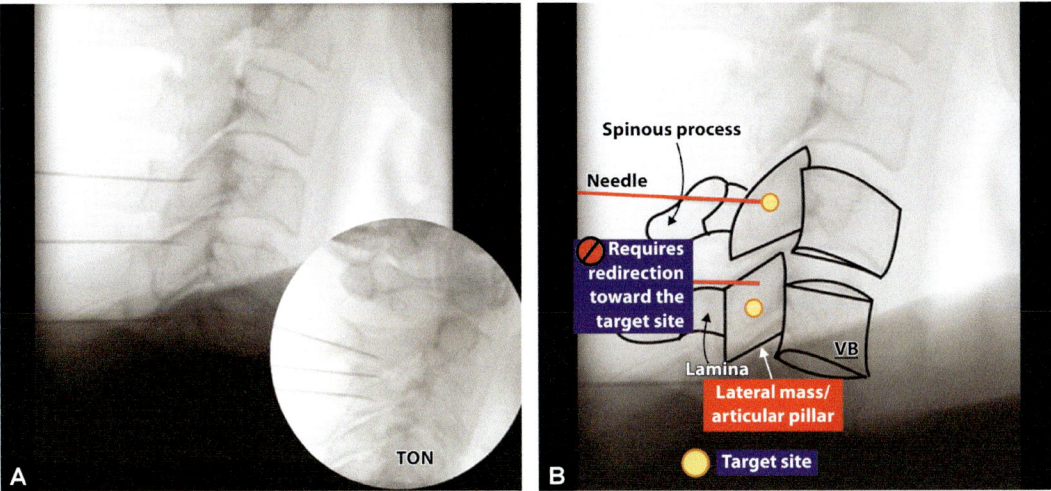

Figs. 3.18A and B: (A) Cervical medial branch block/radiofrequency ablation (RFA) and the third occipital nerve block—lateral view. The needle should be within the midpoint of the "trapezoids" (articular pillar/lateral masses/facet column). Of note, C2 does not have a medial branch but is a potential location of the TON. To block the TON, a needle must be placed at the waist of the C2 and C3 articular pillars and at the C2/C3 facet joint; (B) Cervical medial branch block/RFA—lateral view (labeled).
(TON: Third occipital nerve; VB: Vertebral body).

Injectate
- *Medial branch block*: 0.5 mL of bupivacaine 0.5% at each level.
- *Chemoneurolysis*: 1 mL 50% dextrose or substance of choice.
- *Radiofrequency ablation*: Once complete, administer 1 mL bupivacaine 0.5% with or without 1 mL steroid of choice divided among all the levels.

Techniques
1. *Patient position*: Prone.
2. *Target*: Waists of the articular pillars (where the medial branches lie).
3. *Anteroposterior view*: Square off vertebral body.
   - To improve visualization of the articular pillar waists, tilt caudal 20–30° and rotate ipsilateral 5–10°.
4. Advance spinal needle (3.5–6 inch × 22–25 G) to the inferior portion of the waist of the articular pillar.
5. Contact the "waist" and walk off 2–3 mm.
6. *Lateral view*: Needle should be within the midpoint of the trapezoids/articular pillar/facet column.
7. Confirm placement with a small amount of contrast.
   For RFA, needle placement is identical as above. Before the ablation is carried out, sensory and motor stimulation confirms proximity to medial branch and adequate distance from cervical nerve roots.
8. *Of note*: C2/C3 facet joint is innervated solely by the TON, which is highly variable in location. Hence, blocks are necessary at the C2, C3 waists and the joint line of C2/C3. All three

locations are to target the TON. The C2 nerve root does not give off a dorsal ramus/medial branch.[5]

CERVICAL EPIDURAL STEROID INJECTION (PARASAGITTAL APPROACH) (FIGS. 3.19 TO 3.21)

Indications

- Cervical radiculopathy ± neck pain
- Cervical spinal stenosis
- Treatment of prevention of post herpetic neuralgia.

Advantage

This technique is used to treat multilevel pathology or symptoms which occur bilaterally.

Disadvantages/Complications

- Higher risk of intrathecal injection and cord injury as the width of the cervical epidural space is approximately 3–4 mm, becoming thinner closer toward the head.[3]
- Recommend accessing epidural space at or below C5/C6 interspace and threading up catheter versus achieving adequate spread with volume.
- *Standard epidural steroid injection (ESI) risks*: Unintended dural punctures with PDPH, infection, hematomas, nerve injury, spinal cord infarct, worsening pain, etc.

Injectate

40–80 mg of methylprednisolone or steroid of choice + 1 mL preservative free normal saline (PFNS) + 1 mL bupivacaine 0.25–0.5%.

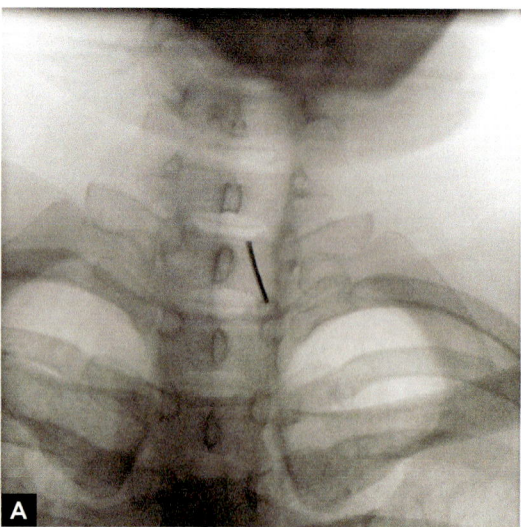 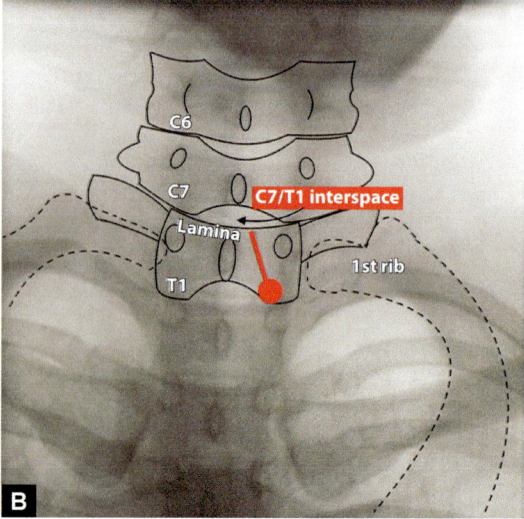

Figs. 3.19A and B: Cervical interlaminar epidural steroid injection (ESI)—anteroposterior (AP) view. To open the interspace, tilt caudally 5–15°. The C7-T1 and T1-2 intervertebral spaces appear to provide a greater margin of safety for cervical epidural punctures. At C7/T1 or T1/T2, the distance from the ligamentum flavum to the dura is 3–5 mm. The width of the epidural space becomes thinner in the higher cervical regions; (B) Cervical interlaminar ESI—AP view. Optional caudal tilt of 5–15° (labeled).

Chapter 3: Head, Neck and Upper Extremity

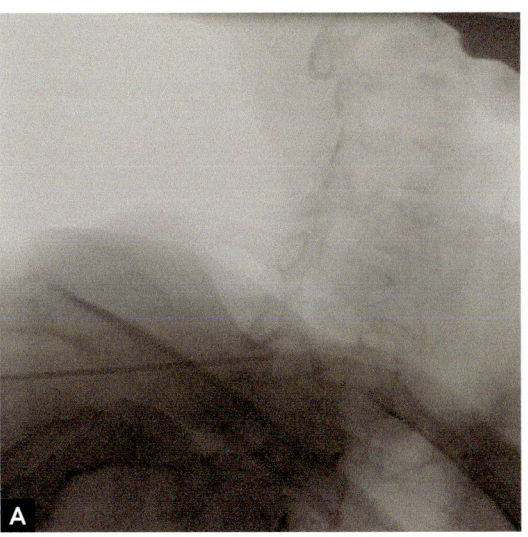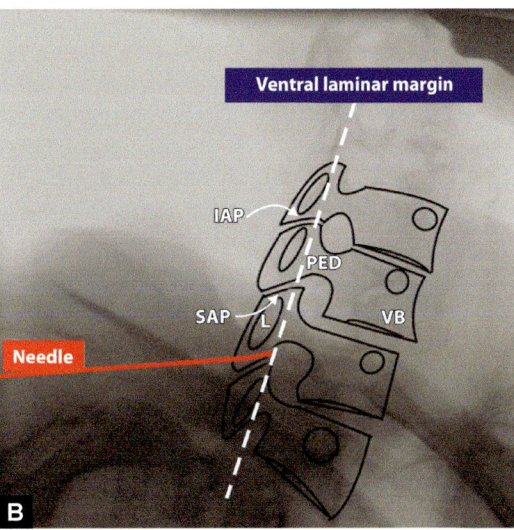

Figs. 3.20A and B: (A) Cervical interlaminar epidural steroid injection (ESI)—contralateral oblique view (50–55°). The needle is advanced to the ventral laminar margin; (B) Cervical interlaminar ESI—contralateral oblique view (50–55°) (labeled).
(IAP: Inferior articular process; SAP: Superior articular process; VB: Vertebral body).

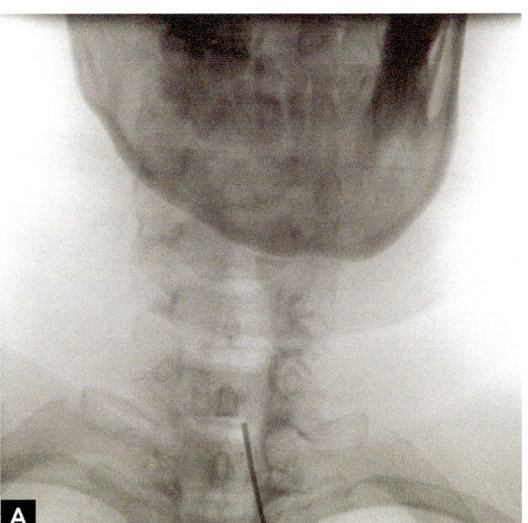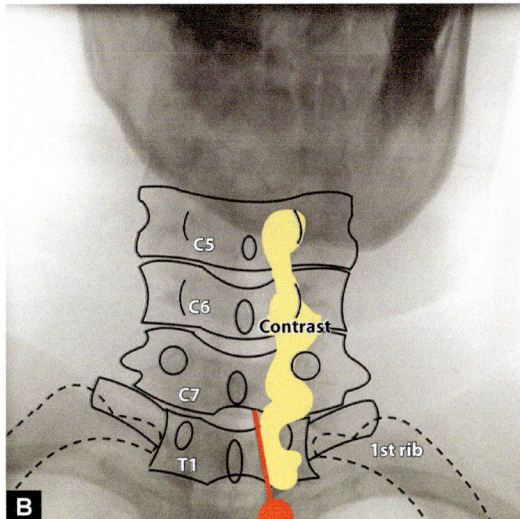

Figs. 3.21A and B: (A) Cervical interlaminar epidural steroid injection (ESI)—anteroposterior (AP) view. Confirmation of contrast spread in the epidural space. [Please see LESI (in Chapter 6) for description on contrast confirmation in the epidural space]; (B) Cervical interlaminar ESI—AP view. Confirmation of contrast spread in the epidural space (labeled).

Techniques

1. *Patient position*: Prone
2. *Anteroposterior view*: Identify the interspace by counting from C1 or T1.

3. *Optimize view*: Tilt caudally 5–15° to open the interspace.
   - If the skull or dentures are obstructing the view, tilt cephalad instead.
4. Advance Tuohy needle (3.5–6 inch × 18–20 G) toward the superior portion of lamina (C7 lamina for C6/C7 interspace) just lateral to midline on the symptomatic side.
5. Contact lamina and step off 2–3 mm.
   - If symptoms are bilateral, direct the needle toward the middle of the interspace.
   - If symptoms are unilateral, angle the needle toward the symptomatic side.
6. Connect the loss of resistance (LOR) syringe and advance until loss.
7. *Contralateral oblique view*: Rotate contralateral 52° to help guide needle advancement. Tip should lie just anterior to the lamina.
8. Confirm placement with contrast in both AP and lateral views.

CERVICAL TRANSFORAMINAL EPIDURAL STEROID INJECTION (FIGS. 3.22 AND 3.23)

Indications
- Cervical radiculopathy with or without neck pain
- Cervical spinal stenosis.

Advantages
- Technique can also be used for diagnostic selective nerve root block.
- Technique can also be used for cervical discography (beyond the scope of this book).
- It can be performed with minimal risk using proper technique, digital subtraction angiography (DSA) and non-particulate steroids.

Disadvantages/Complications
- Highest risk for intravascular injection (vertebral artery most frequently ventral to nerve but occasionally behind nerve, radicular branches above or ventral to nerve).

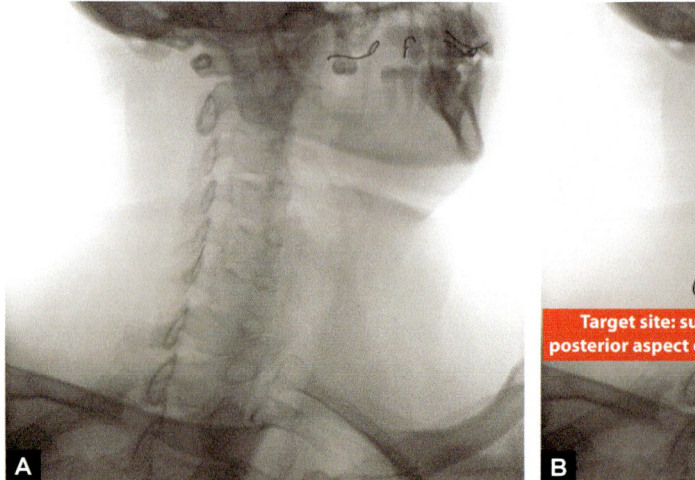
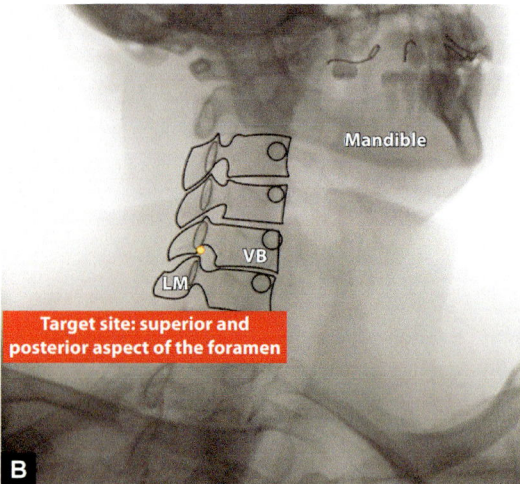

Figs. 3.22A and B: (A) Cervical transforaminal epidural steroid injection (ESI)—foraminal view (45° ipsilateral rotation) with a caudal tilt of 5–10° to square off the vertebral body end plates; (B) Cervical transforaminal ESI—foraminal view (labeled).

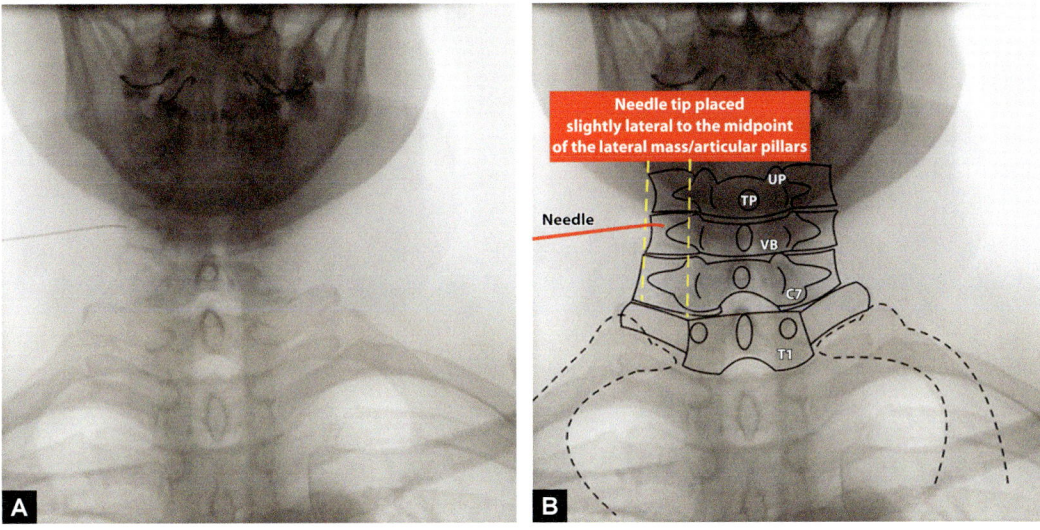

Figs. 3.23A and B: (A) Cervical transforaminal epidural steroid injection (ESI)—anteroposterior (AP) view. Advance the needle to the midpoint of the lateral masses/articular pillars; (B) Cervical transforaminal ESI—PA view (labeled).

- Direct trauma to the nerve root (sits immediately anterior to SAP).
- *Standard ESI risks*: Infection, hematomas, subarachnoid injection, intrathecal injection, spinal cord injury, nerve injury, spinal cord infarct, worsening pain, etc.

Injectate
- 4–8 mg of dexamethasone + 1 mL PFNS.
- Local anesthetics are typically avoided for safety reasons.

Techniques
1. *Patient position*: Supine
2. *Target*: Sagittal midline of articular pillars in foramen, medial to uncinate process.
3. *Foraminal view*: Rotate ipsilateral 45° (40–50°), square off the end plates by tilting caudal 5–10°.
    - Adjust further until foramen is maximally tall and wide without encroachment.
    - *Caution*: Medial foramen is smaller in diameter than the lateral border so hug outer border with needle tip to avoid accidental entrance into the central canal.
4. Advance spinal needle (3.5 inch × 22–25 G) toward the portion of the posterior edge of the foramen (larger, more posterior border).
5. Contact the SAP
6. *Posteroanterior view*: Advance needle in this position 2–3 mm until the tip lies at the midpoint of the articular pillars and never past the uncinate process (risks puncturing thecal sac).
7. Confirm placement with contrast under live fluoroscopy in AP and lateral views. Highly recommend DSA when available.

SPINAL CORD STIMULATOR TRIAL—CERVICAL (FIGS. 3.24 AND 3.25)

Indications
- Patients who have failed interventions and conservative management.
- Cervical radiculopathy ± axial neck pain, complex regional pain syndrome, painful peripheral neuropathies, brachial plexopathy.
- Failed "neck" syndrome.

Advantages
- Direct stimulation of the dorsal column can cause changes within the ascending sensory fibers that modulate the intensity of painful stimuli.
- Potential for long-term benefits.
- Steroid sparing.

Disadvantages/Complications
- Lead migration, lead fracture, and discomfort with paresthesia.
- *Standard ESI risks*: Unintended dural puncture with PDPH, infection, hematomas, nerve injury, spinal cord infarct, worsening pain, etc.

Injectate
None

Techniques
1. *Pre-procedure*: Administer antibiotics (i.e. IV cefazolin 2 g).
2. *Patient position*: Prone with pillows under the abdomen to minimize lordosis.

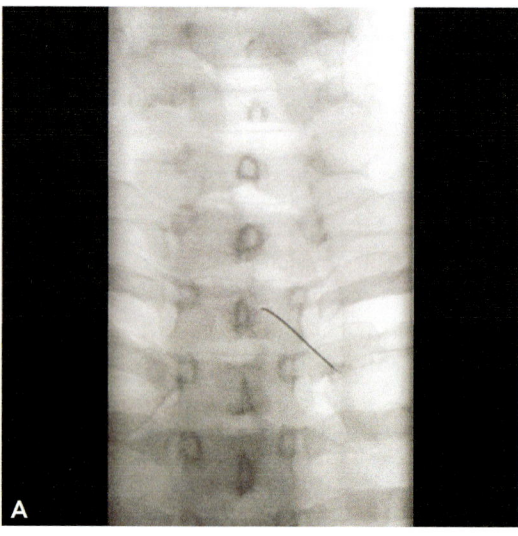 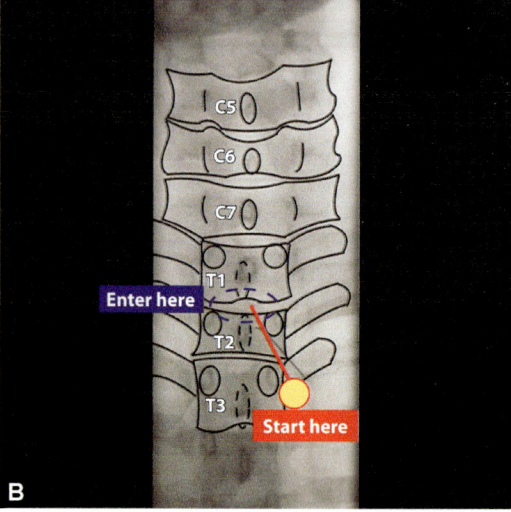

Figs. 3.24A and B: (A) Cervical spinal cord stimulator trial—anteroposterior (AP) view. Target the T1/T2 or the T2/T3 interspace. To enter the interspace at a 45° angle, place the epidural introducer needle just lateral to the pedicle one level below the level of entrance (approximate 20–30° angle from midline). This directs the lead midline upon epidural access and the shallow angle facilitates lead steering; (B) Cervical spinal cord stimulator trial—AP view (labeled).

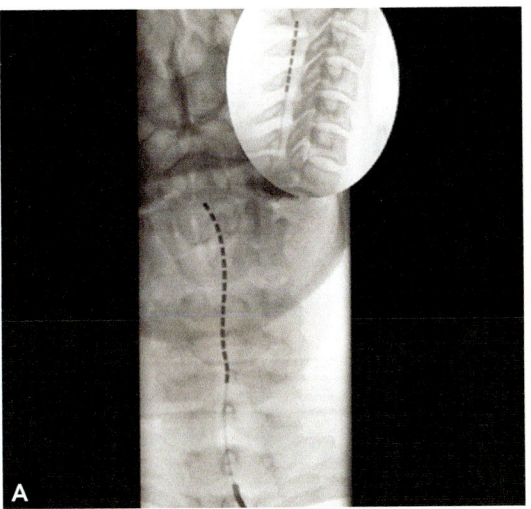 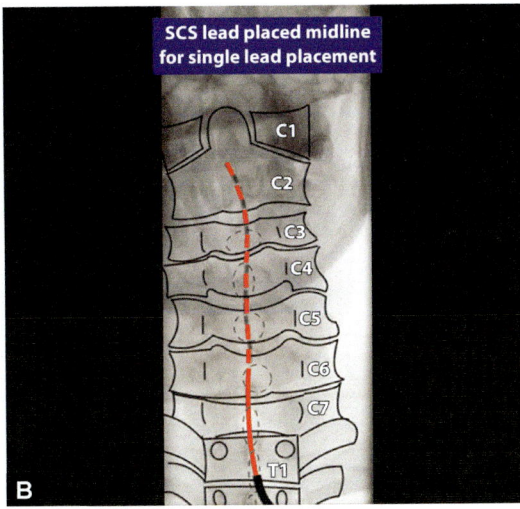

Figs. 3.25A and B: Cervical spinal cord stimulator trial—anteroposterior (AP) and lateral view. Lead placement; (B) Cervical spinal cord stimulator trial—AP view (labeled). (SCS: Spinal cord stimulator).

3. *Target*: C7/T1, T1/T2, or T2/T3 epidural interspace.
4. *Anteroposterior view*: Square off the respective vertebral body and ensure spinous process is midline.
   - Tilt caudally 5–15° to open up the interspace.
5. Start by placing the epidural introducer needle just lateral to the pedicle one level below the level of entrance (approximate 20–30° angle from midline). This directs the lead midline upon epidural access and the shallow angle facilitates lead steering.
   - Advance toward midline of the targeted interspace.
   - The needle should be advanced at a 30–45° angle from the skin
6. Contact the edge of the lamina and walk off:
   - Connect LOR syringe to needle
   - Advance toward midline until LOR occurs.
7. Thread lead through the introducer needle and advance lead *midline* (See table for lead placement).[4]

Cervical lead placement	Painful areas
C2	Head (V2 or V3 distribution)
C2 to C4	Neck, shoulder, arm
C4 to C7	Forearm to hand
C7 to T1	Anterior shoulder

8. *Lateral view*: Confirm placement in posterior epidural space.
9. Adjust leads based on stimulation test.
10. A second parallel lead may be required if pain is bilateral and not covered by a single lead. If so, the leads should be placed 2–3 mm lateral on each side of midline.

34 *Fluoro-Flip: A Quick Reference Guide to Spinal and Peripheral Pain Procedures*

STELLATE GANGLION BLOCK (FIGS. 3.26 AND 3.27)

Indication
Sympathetically mediated pain conditions of the head, neck and upper extremity such as CRPS, phantom limb pain, or neuropathic pain.

Advantage
Provides diagnostic and therapeutic value.

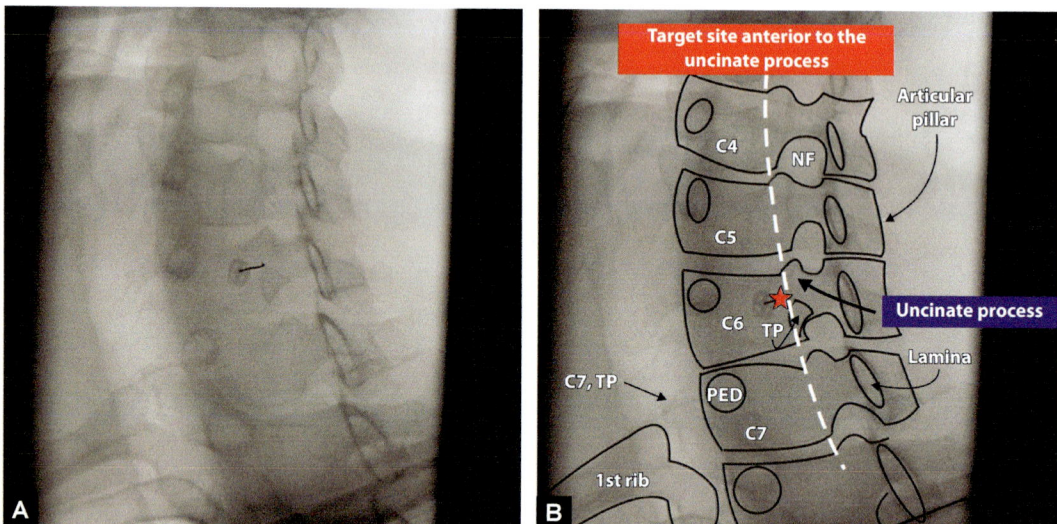

Figs. 3.26A and B: (A) Stellate ganglion block—foraminal view; (B) Stellate ganglion block—foraminal view (labeled).

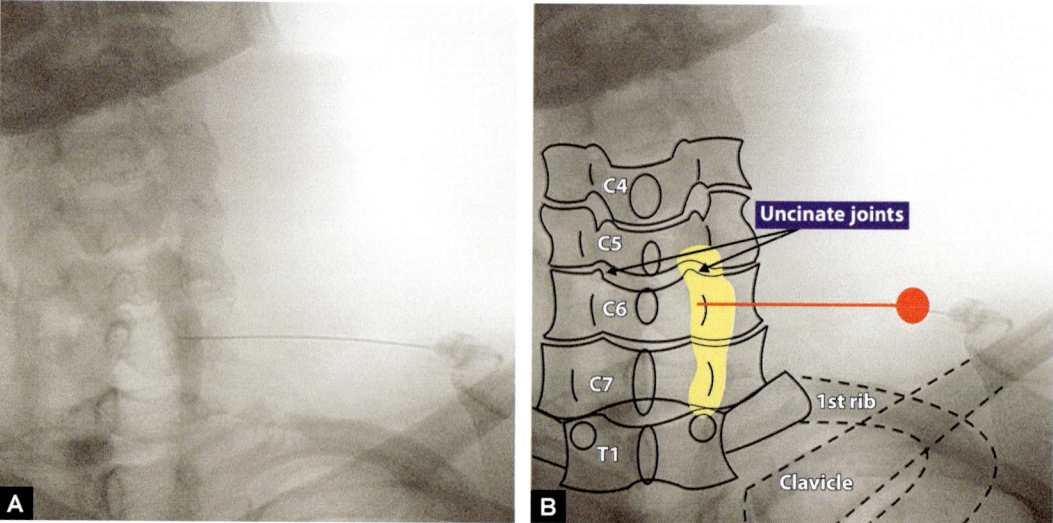

Figs. 3.27A and B: (A) Stellate ganglion block—posteroanterior (PA) view. Contrast spread along the longus colli muscle; (B) Stellate ganglion block—PA view (labeled).

Disadvantages/Complications
- Higher risk for pneumothorax, intravascular injection (carotid and vertebral arteries) at C7 level, hence the procedure is performed at the C6 level.
- There are a small number of somatic branches from the second thoracic spinal nerve termed "Kuntz's fibers" which bypass the stellate ganglion. This can result in an incomplete sympathetic blockade. A brachial plexus block would be able to block the "Kuntz's fibers" however would not be selective for sympathetic fibers.
- Bilateral injections should not be performed as blocking bilateral recurrent laryngeal and/or phrenic nerves may result in respiratory failure and hoarseness.

Injectate
4–8 mg of Decadron or steroid of choice with 10 mL of bupivacaine 0.5%.

Techniques
1. *Patient position*: Supine, head slightly extended.
2. *Target*: Inferior portion of the uncinate process at the junction of the transverse process (TP) (Chassaignac's tubercle) and the vertebral body.
3. *Posteroanterior view*: Identify the C6 vertebral body and Chassaignac's tubercle.
4. *Oblique view*: Rotate ipsilateral 40–45° to allow adequate visualization of the neural foramina. This trajectory avoids the more medially located neurovascular structures.
5. Advance spinal needle (3.5 inch × 22–25 G) coaxially toward the target:
   - Be cautious to avoid entering the neural foramina
   - Contact the surface of the vertebral body at the target junction as described above.
6. Confirm placement with contrast and live fluoroscopy.
7. A sympathetic block should be noted within 20 minutes (i.e. Horner's syndrome, increase in temperature by 1–2°C in the ipsilateral upper extremity). If temperature change is achieved however no pain relief, patient's pain may be sympathetically independent.

GLENOHUMERAL SHOULDER INTRA-ARTICULAR INJECTION (ANTERIOR APPROACH) (FIGS. 3.28 AND 3.29)

Indication
Shoulder pain, shoulder osteoarthritis.

Advantage
Safe and accurate placement of steroids compared to blind or ultrasound-guided technique.

Disadvantages/Complications
- Neurovascular injection
- Multiple steroid injections can have deleterious effect on cartilage, cause bone loss, osteoporosis, and osteonecrosis.
- Infection

Injectate
40 mg of methylprednisolone or steroid of choice + 3–4 mL of bupivacaine 0.25–0.5%.

Techniques
1. *Patient position*: Supine

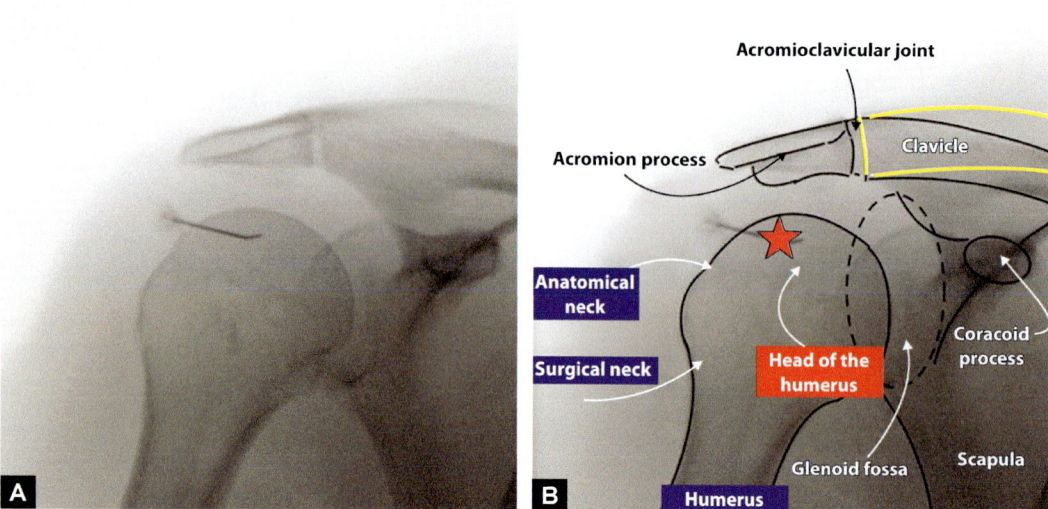

Figs. 3.28A and B: (A) Glenohumeral intra-articular injection—posteroanterior (PA) view. Target the superolateral portion of the humeral head; (B) Glenohumeral intra-articular injection—PA view (labeled).

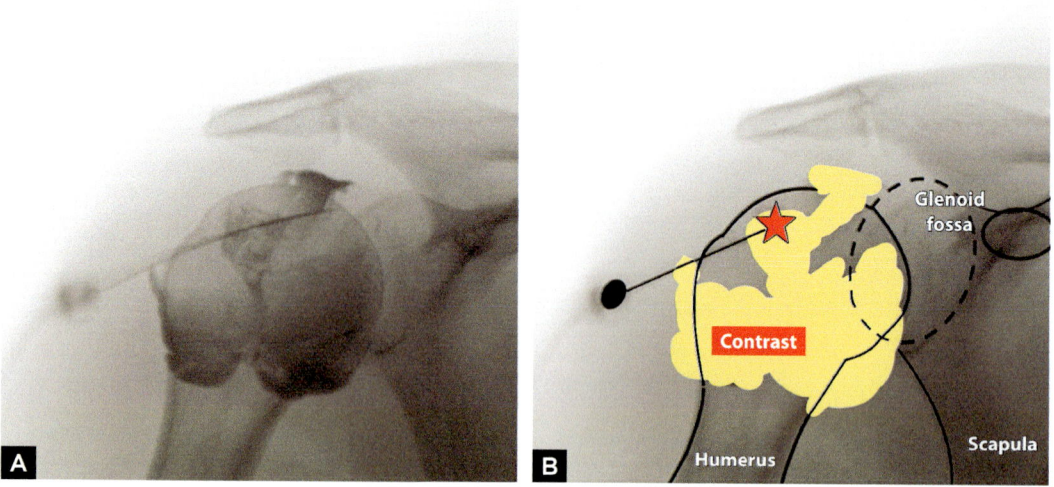

Figs. 3.29A and B: (A) Glenohumeral intra-articular injection—posteroanterior (PA) view. Contrast spread within the joint; (B) Glenohumeral intra-articular injection—PA view. Contrast spread within the joint (labeled).

2. *Target*: Superolateral portion of the humeral head (lateral one-third of the humeral head).
3. *Anteroposterior view*: Identify the humeral head.
4. Advance spinal needle (3.5 inch × 22–25 G) toward target until humerus is contact.
5. Confirm placement with contrast. The arthrogram should display a circumferential spread.

REFERENCES

1. Murthy NS, Maus TP, Aprill C. The retrodural space of Okada. AJR Am J Roentgenol. 2011;196(6):W784-9.
2. Okada K. Studies on the cervical facet joints using arthrography of the cervical facet joint (author's transl). Nihon Seikeigeka Gakkai Zasshi. 1981;55(6):563-80.
3. Aldrete JA, Mushin AU, Zapata JC, et al. Skin to cervical epidural space distances as read from magnetic resonance imaging films: consideration of the "hump pad." J Clin Anesth. 1998;10(4):309-13.
4. Deer TR. Atlas of Implantable Therapies for Pain Management. New York: Springer Science+Business Media; 2010.
5. Lord SM, Barnsley L, Bogduk N. Percutaneous radiofrequency neurotomy in the treatment of cervical zygapophysial joint pain: a caution. Neurosurgery. 1995;36(4):732-9.

Chapter 4

Thoracic, Chest and Abdomen

THORACIC INTRA-ARTICULAR FACET INJECTION (FIGS. 4.1 TO 4.3)

Indications
- Thoracic spondylosis
- Mid axial back pain without radicular symptoms.

Advantages
- Intra-articular injections are diagnostic and therapeutic interventions.
- With enough volume, injectate can also achieve epidural spread and indirectly provide similar benefits to an epidural steroid injection (ESI).

Disadvantages/Complications
- Difficult to visualize on fluoroscopy (no optimal angle)
- Worsening pain, pneumothorax, epidural spread if volume of injectate is more than 1.5 mL, spinal cord injury.

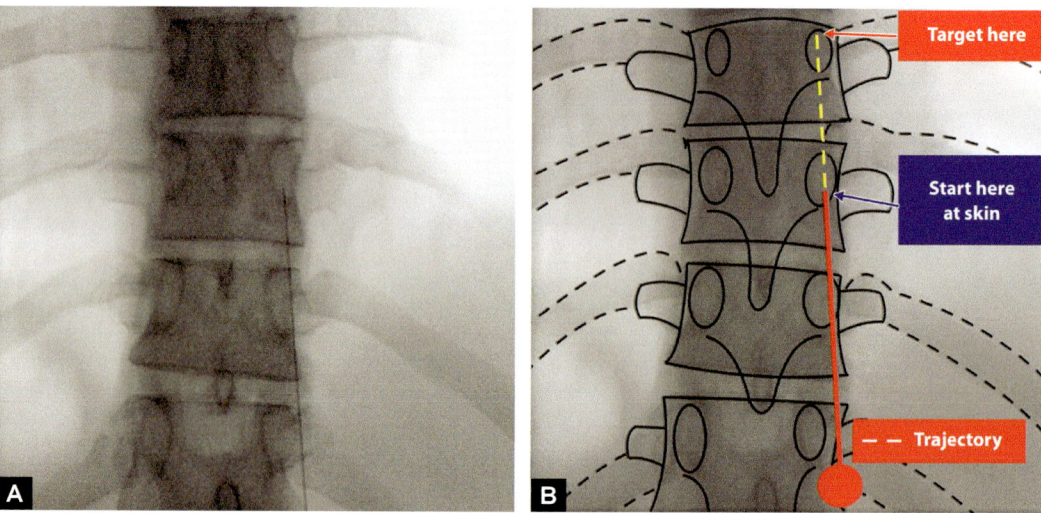

Figs. 4.1A and B: (A) Thoracic facet intra-articular injection—anteroposterior (AP) view. Start at the pedicle at the vertebral body below the targeted facet joint. Insert the needle at a 45–60° angle toward the facet joint. Use a contralateral oblique view for needle advancement; (B) Thoracic facet intra-articular injection–AP view (labeled).

Chapter 4: Thoracic, Chest and Abdomen

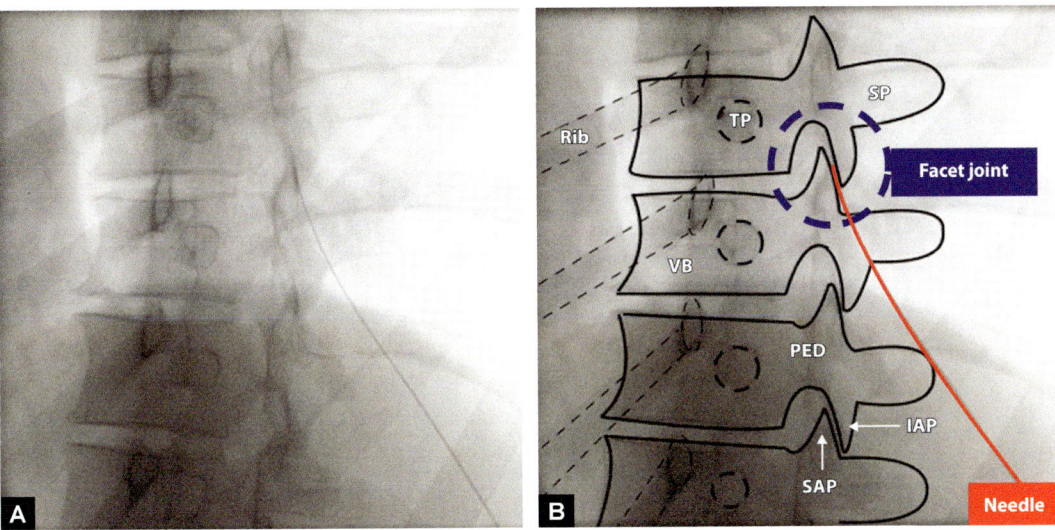

Figs. 4.2A and B: (A) Thoracic facet intra-articular injection—contralateral oblique view (50–55°). Needle is advanced toward the facet joint; (B) Thoracic facet intra-articular injection—contralateral oblique view (labeled). (SP: Spinous process; TP: Transverse process; VB: Vertebral body; PED: Pedicle; IAP: Inferior articular process; SAP: Superior articular process).

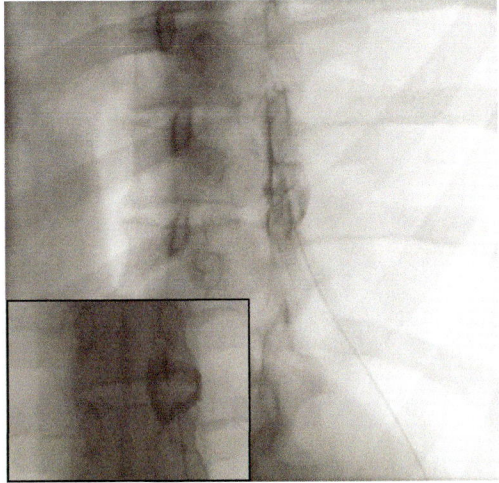

Fig. 4.3: Thoracic facet intra-articular injection—contralateral oblique and anteroposterior (AP) view of contrast spread.

Injectate

0.5–1 mL of 40–80 mg of methylprednisolone or steroid of choice + bupivacaine 0.5% divided among the joints.

Techniques

1. *Patient position*: Prone
2. *Target*: Inferior portion of the facet.

3. *Anteroposterior view*: Identify pedicle at the vertebral body below the targeted facet joint (i.e. the pathologic facet is at the T6/T7; your needle entry will be at the 6 o'clock position of the T8 pedicle). This allows a shallow trajectory which facilitates walking into the facet.
4. Advance needle at approximately 60° toward the superior portion of the pedicle above at approximately 12 o'clock position (i.e. target T7 for T6/T7 joint).
5. Contact lamina and turn needle tip superiorly.
6. *Contralateral oblique view*: Advance needle in this view into the joint.
7. Confirm placement with contrast in anteroposterior (AP) and lateral views.

THORACIC MEDIAL BRANCH BLOCK AND RADIOFREQUENCY ABLATION (FIGS. 4.4 TO 4.6)

Indications
- Thoracic spondylosis
- Facet arthrosis
- Axial back pain without radicular symptoms.

Advantages
- Medial branch block (MBB) provides diagnostic information.
- Chemoneurolytic ablation can be easily done using the MBB technique and by administering a chemoneurolytic substance (phenol, methylene blue, 50% dextrose).
- Radiofrequency ablation (RFA) provides longer lasting relief.

Disadvantages/Complications
- Variable location of the medial branch (MB) in the thoracic region.
- Diagnostic blocks provide short-term duration (<12 hours if only bupivacaine is used).

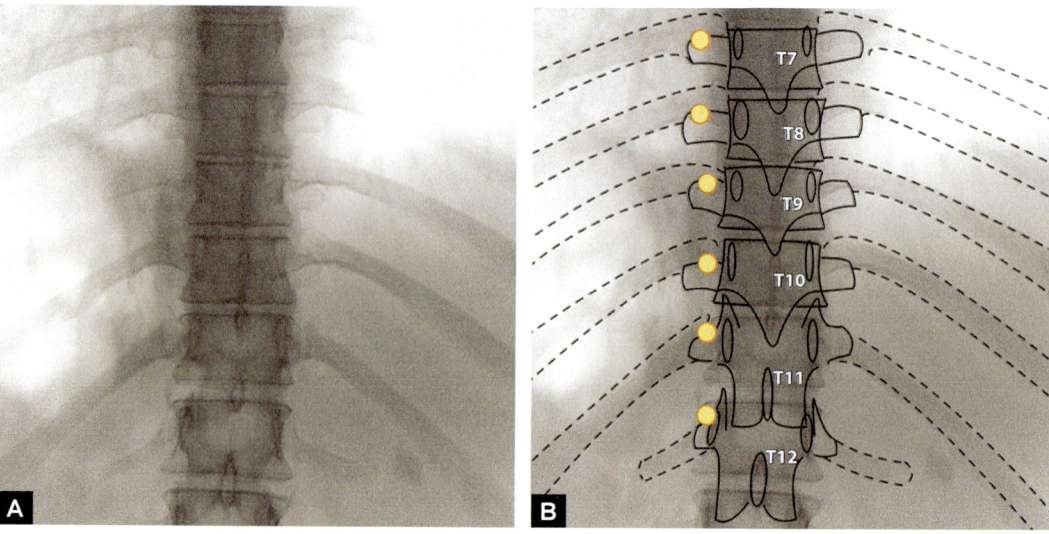

Figs. 4.4A and B: (A) Thoracic medial branch blocks—anteroposterior (AP) view; (B) Thoracic medial branch block—AP view. Target points (labeled).

Chapter 4: Thoracic, Chest and Abdomen

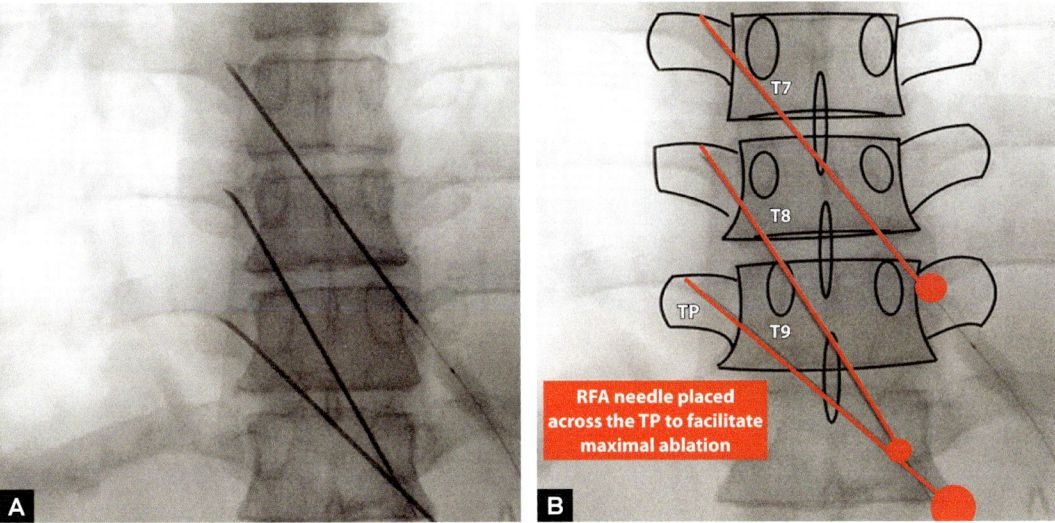

Figs. 4.5A and B: (A) Thoracic medial branch block (MBB)/radiofrequency ablation (RFA)—anteroposterior (AP) view; (B) Thoracic MBB/RFA—AP view (labeled). (TP: Transverse process).

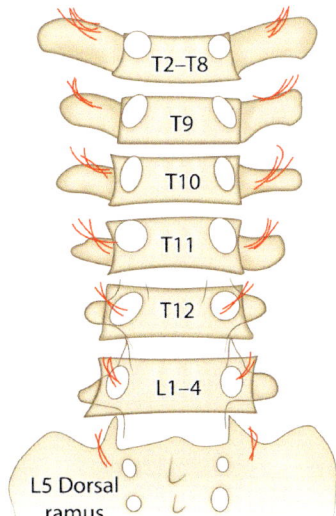

Fig. 4.6: Anatomic location of the thoracic medial branch.[1]

- Minimal sedatives can falsify diagnostic information (i.e. giving midazolam causes muscle relaxation, and fentanyl can diminish pain scores).
- Requires multiple levels of injections as each joint is innervated by the medial branch at the level and the level above the joint (i.e. L4-5 joint by L3 MB and L4 MB).

Injectate
- *Medial branch block*: 0.5 mL of bupivacaine 0.5% at each level.
- *Chemoneurolysis*: 1 mL 50% dextrose or substance of choice.

- *Radiofrequency ablation*: Once complete, administer 1 mL bupivacaine 0.5% with or without 1 mL steroid of choice divided among all the levels.

Techniques
1. *Patient position*: Prone
2. *Target*:
   - ◊ T1-T10: Superolateral edge of the transverse process (TP).
   - ◊ T11, T12: Superior articular process (SAP) and TP junction (same as lumbar MBB).
3. *Anteroposterior view*: Square off vertebral body at the level of the injection:
   - ◊ Advance spinal needle (3.5-6 inch × 22-25 G) and contact TP at the target site.
4. *Lateral view*: Walk off superiorly 1-2 mm.
5. For MBB, confirm placement with a small amount of contrast.
6. *For RFA*:
   - ◊ Needle entry should be at the bisection of the mid vertebral body level and the middle of the pedicle. This facilitates maximal ablation tip surface area contact with the medial branch.
   - ◊ Before the ablation is carried out, sensory and motor stimulation confirms proximity to medial branch yet away from the spinal nerve. Needle may need to be adjusted based upon stimulation given the variable locations of the thoracic medial branches.

THORACIC EPIDURAL STEROID INJECTION (PARASAGITTAL APPROACH) (FIGS. 4.7 AND 4.8)

Indications
- Thoracic radiculopathy ± axial back pain
- Thoracic spinal stenosis
- Treatment or prevention of postherpetic neuralgia.

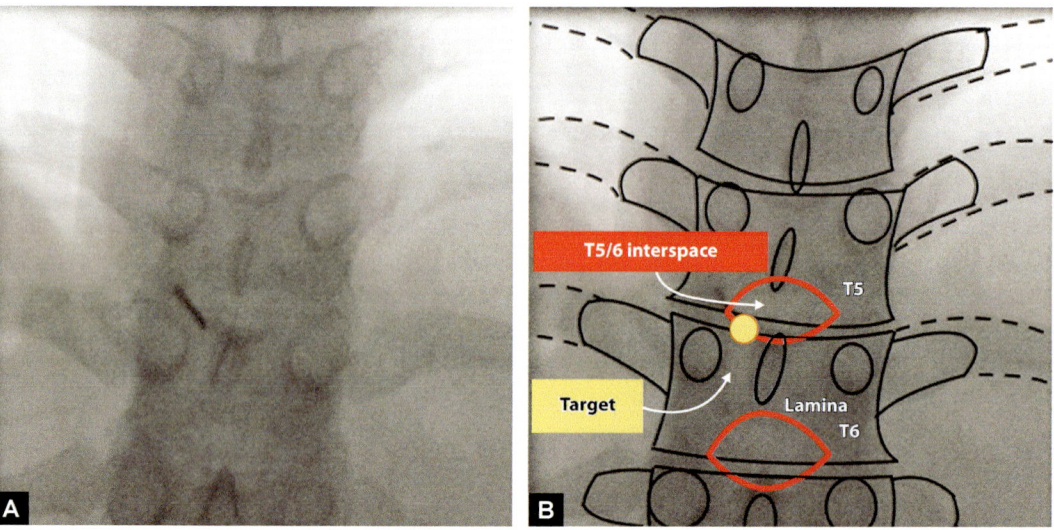

Figs. 4.7A and B: (A) Thoracic interlaminar epidural steroid injection (ESI)—anteroposterior (AP) view with a caudal tilt of 25–35° to "open" the interspace; (B) Thoracic interlaminar ESI—AP view with a caudal tilt of 25–35° (labeled).

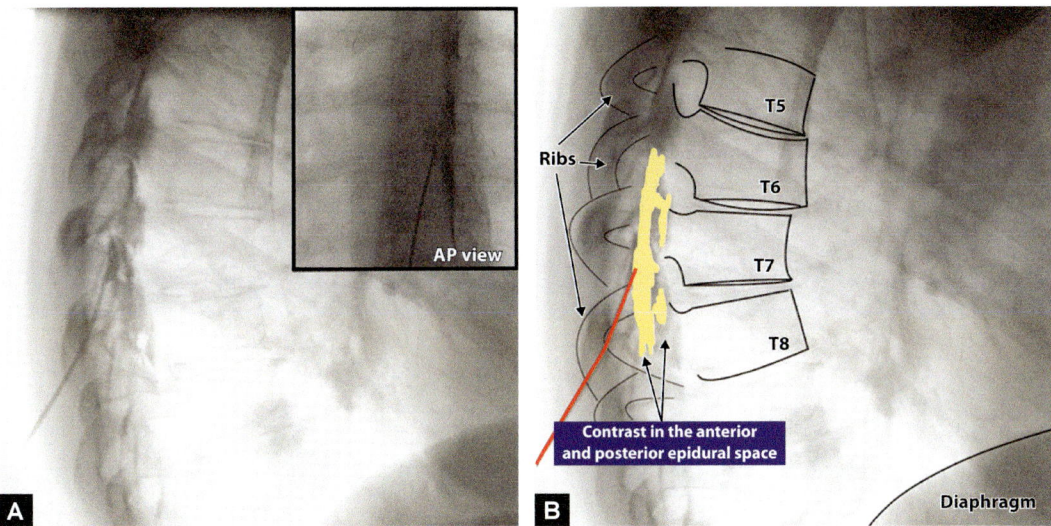

Figs. 4. 8A and B: (A) Thoracic interlaminar epidural steroid injection (ESI)—lateral view and anteroposterior (AP) view. Contrast spread; (B) Thoracic interlaminar ESI—lateral view. Contrast spread (labeled).

Advantages
Treats multilevel pathology and bilateral symptoms.

Disadvantages/Complications
Standard ESI risks: Spinal cord injury, unintended dural puncture with post-dural puncture headache (PDPH), infection, hematomas, nerve injury, spinal cord infarct, worsening pain, etc.

Injectate
40–80 mg of methylprednisolone or steroid of choice + 1 mL PFNS + 1 mL bupivacaine 0.25–0.5%.

Techniques
1. *Patient position*: Prone
2. *Target*: Interspace just lateral to midline on the symptomatic side.
3. *Anteroposterior view*: Square off vertebral body at target level, identify interspace.
4. *Optimize view*: Tilt caudally 25–35° or until the interspaces open.
5. Advance Tuohy needle (3.5–6 inch × 18–20 G) toward the superior portion of the lamina (i.e. contact T9 lamina for T8/T9 interspace) just lateral to midline on the symptomatic side.
6. Contact lamina and step off 2–3 mm:
   ◊ If symptoms are bilateral, direct the needle toward the middle of the interspace
   ◊ If symptoms are unilateral, angle the needle toward the symptomatic side.
7. Connect to the loss of resistance (LOR) syringe and advance until loss is encountered.
8. *Contralateral oblique view*: Rotate contralateral 52°
   ◊ Needle tip should be just anterior to the lamina
9. Confirm needle placement with contrast in both AP and lateral views.

INTERCOSTAL NERVE BLOCKS (FIGS. 4.9A AND B)

Indications
- Chest wall pain, rib fractures, thoracic neuropathic pain, and abdominal pain
- Intercostal neuralgia due to breast or cardiac surgery
- Postherpetic neuralgia pain.

Advantage
Provides both diagnostic and therapeutic value with potential to proceed to RFA for sustained relief.

Disadvantages/Complications
- Pneumothorax
- Intravascular injection (remember "VAN" from superior to inferior-vein, artery, nerve)
- Risk for local toxicity (higher rate for absorption: intercostal blocks > epidural/caudal > brachial plexus and femoral/sciatic nerve blocks > subcutaneous injections).

Injectate
2–4 mL of 40–80 mg of methylprednisolone or steroid of choice + bupivacaine 0.5% divided among total injections.

Techniques
1. Place the patient in the prone position.
2. *Target*: Inferior intercostal margin of rib.
3. *Anteroposterior view*: Squaring off vertebral body will require tilting caudal 15–20°.

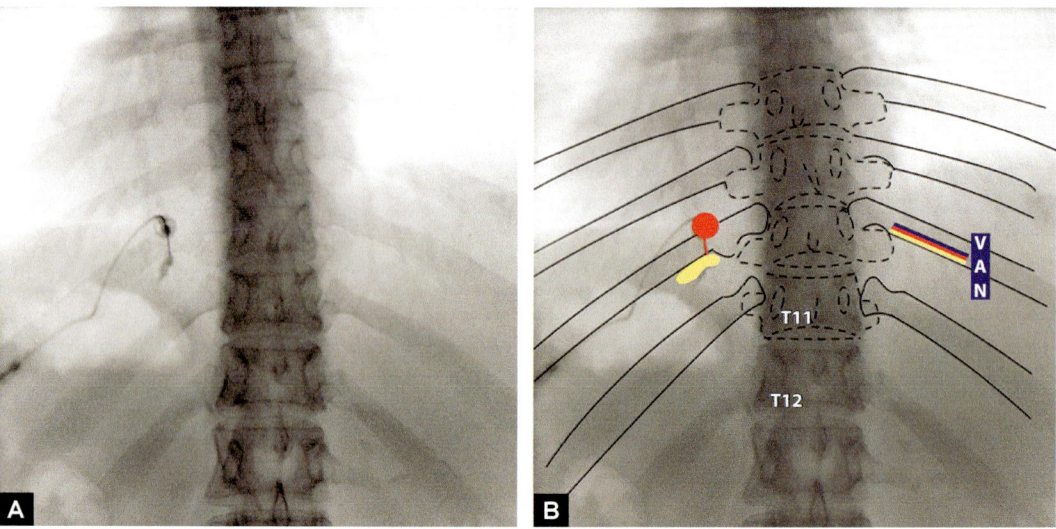

Figs. 4.9A and B: (A) Intercostal block—anteroposterior (AP) view with a caudal tilt of 15–20°; (B) Intercostal block—AP view with a caudal tilt of 15–20° (labeled).

4. Advance needle (1.5-3.5 inch × 22-25 G) needle 1.5-3.5-inch needle toward target:
   ◊ To maximize portion of nerve blocked, tip should be no more lateral than the medial scapular border or 3-4 inches lateral to the spinous process.
5. Contact inferior intercostal margin with needle and walk off 2-3 mm.
6. *Lateral view*: Determine depth.
7. Confirm placement with contrast:
   ◊ Contrast should flow along the intercostal margin
   ◊ A striated pattern suggests intramuscular injection. Advance needle 1-3 mm.

SPLANCHNIC NERVE BLOCK (RETROCRURAL TECHNIQUE) (FIGS. 4.10 TO 4.12)

Indications
Treatment of abdominal visceral pain such as that related to the pancreas, liver, gallbladder, and the alimentary tract from the stomach to the transverse colon.

Advantages
- Compared to celiac plexus blocks, splanchnic nerve block avoids the risk of aortic penetration.
- No evidence that splanchnic nerve blocks are inferior to celiac plexus blocks.

Disadvantages/Complications
- High risk for pneumothorax.
- When blocks are bilateral, higher risk of hypotension and diarrhea as side effects.
- Epidural/Intrathecal block.

Injectate
40-80 mg of methylprednisolone or steroid of choice per side + 10 mL of bupivacaine 0.25-0.5%.

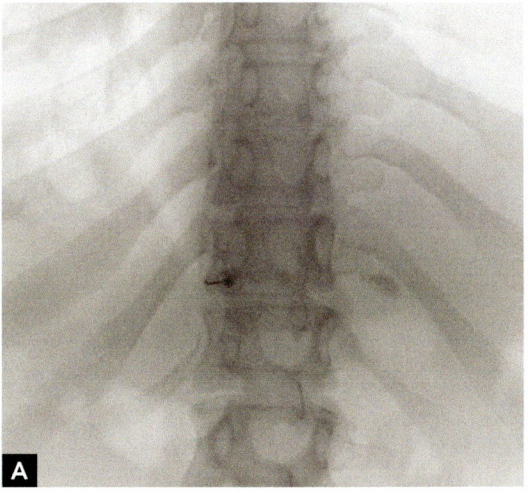
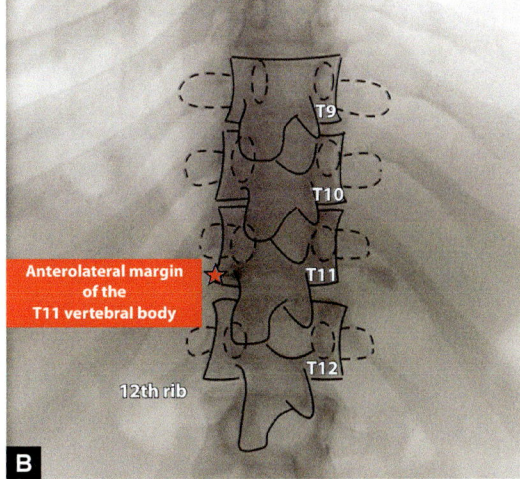

Figs. 4.10A and B: (A) Splanchnic nerve block—anteroposterior (AP) view with a 5-10° ipsilateral rotation. A rotation greater than 10° may increase the risk of a pneumothorax; (B) Splanchnic nerve block—AP view with a 5-10° ipsilateral rotation (labeled).

46 Fluoro-Flip: A Quick Reference Guide to Spinal and Peripheral Pain Procedures

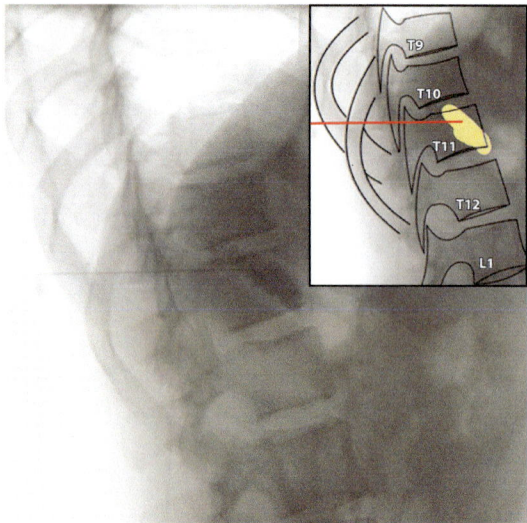

Fig. 4.11: Splanchnic nerve block—lateral view. Needle placed at the two-thirds anterolateral margin of the T11 vertebral body. Contrast spread.

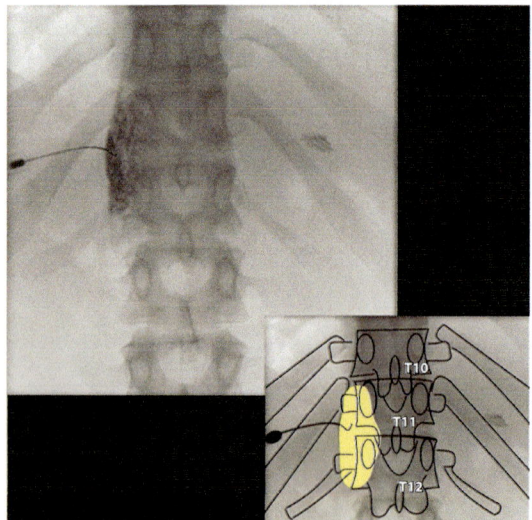

Fig. 4.12: Splanchnic nerve block—anteroposterior (AP) view. Contrast spread.

Techniques
1. *Patient position*: Prone
2. *Target*: Anterior two-thirds of the lateral margin of the T11 or T12 vertebral body.
3. *Anteroposterior view*: Square off the vertebral body.
    ◊ Rotate ipsilateral 5–10° until the anterior portion of the vertebral body is visible.
    ◊ If rib is overlying the target, tilt caudal.
4. Advance spinal needle (5–6 inch × 22 G) toward the target.

5. *Lateral view*: Obtain periodically to determine the depth.
   ◊ Once contact is made with vertebral body, advance in lateral view until needle tip is at target as described above.
   ◊ Maintain osseous contact with the vertebral body wall to avoid straying too lateral.
6. Confirm placement with contrast in AP and lateral views.

CELIAC PLEXUS BLOCK (TRANSCRURAL TECHNIQUE) (FIGS. 4.13 TO 4.15)

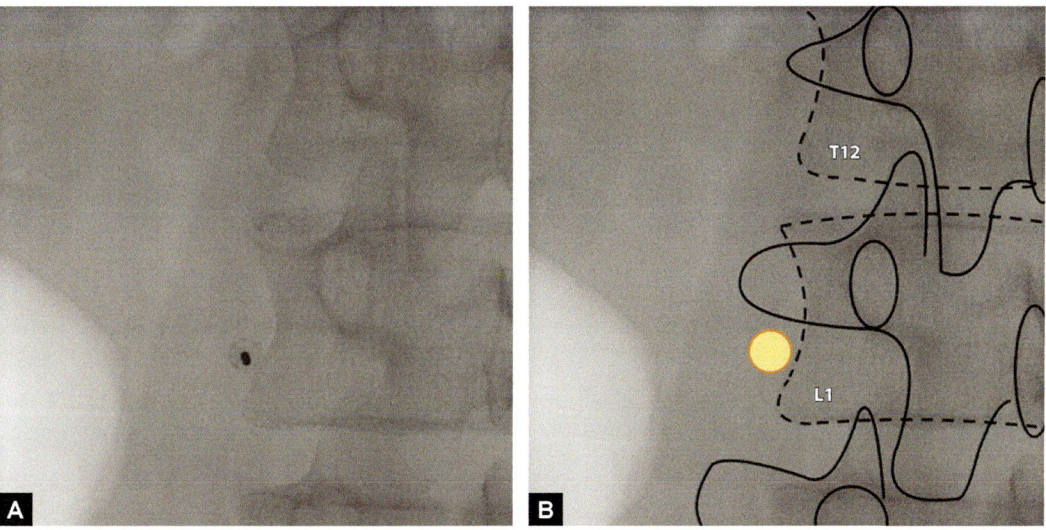

Figs. 4.13A and B: (A) Celiac plexus block—20–30° ipsilateral rotation or until the transverse process is at the anterolateral margin of the vertebral margin; (B) Celiac plexus block—20–30° ipsilateral rotation (labeled).

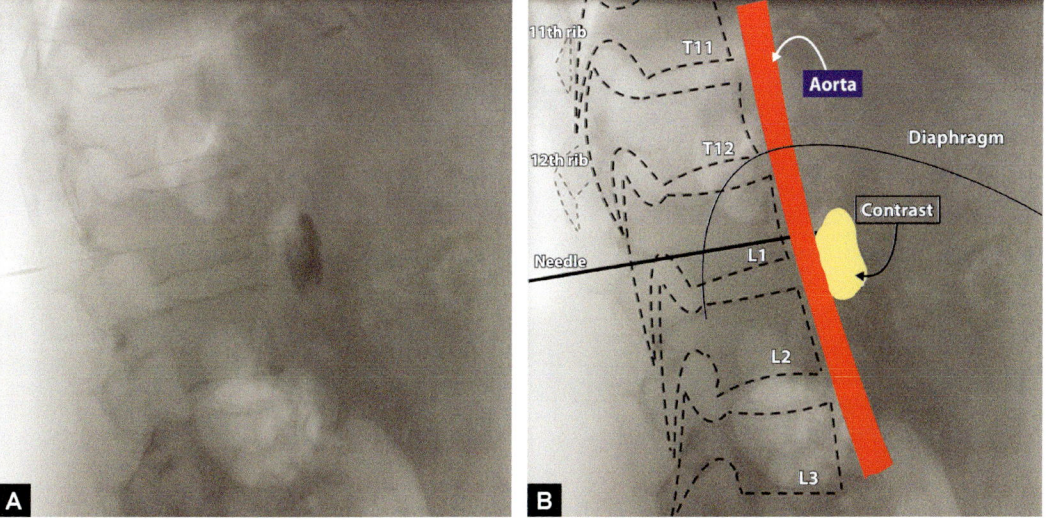

Figs. 4.14A and B: (A) Celiac plexus block—lateral view. Contrast spread anterior to the aorta; (B) Celiac plexus block—lateral view. Contrast spread anterior to the aorta (labeled).

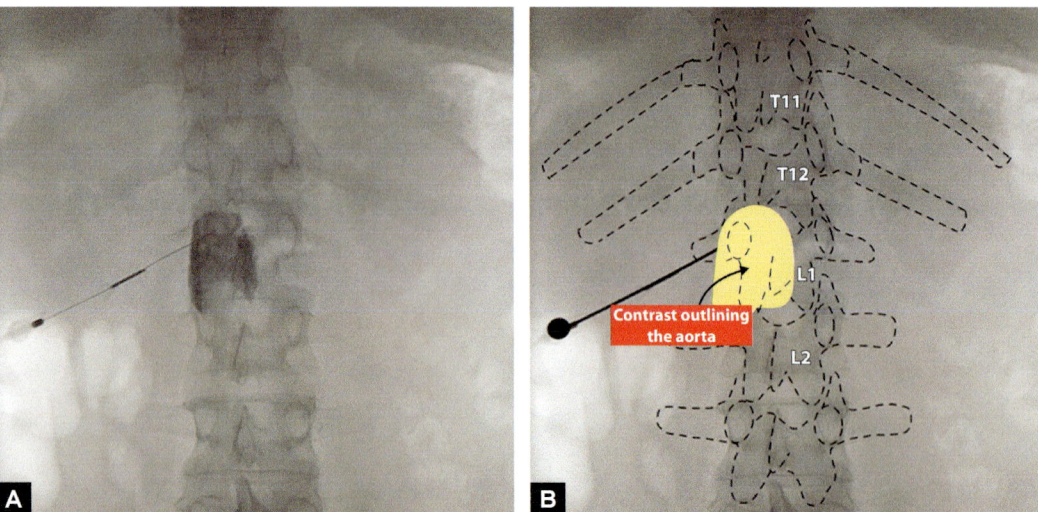

Figs. 4.15A and B: (A) Celiac plexus block—anteroposterior (AP) view. Contrast spread outlining anterior and anterolateral to the aorta; (B) Celiac plexus block—AP view. Contrast spread in the celiac region (anterolateral wall of the aorta, anterior to the crura of the diaphragm, from above the celiac artery to the superior mesenteric artery)-labeled.

Indication

Treatment of abdominal visceral pain such as that related to the pancreas, liver, gallbladder, and the alimentary tract from the stomach to the transverse colon.

Advantages

- A single needle can be used for bilateral treatment compared to the splanchnic nerve block which requires bilateral injections
- Neurolysis can be performed for prolonged relief.

Disadvantages/Complications

- High risk for pneumothorax, hypotension, and diarrhea.
- Epidural/Intrathecal block

Injectate

40–80 mg of methylprednisolone or steroid of choice + 10 mL of bupivacaine 0.25–0.5%.

Techniques

1. *Patient position*: Prone
2. *Target*: 2–3 cm past the superior edge of the L1 vertebral body.
3. *Anteroposterior view*: Rotate left 20–30° or until the TP is at the anterolateral margin of the vertebral body (the ganglia is anterior to the aorta and lies to the left side).
4. Advance spinal needle (5–6 inch × 22–25 G) toward the target.
5. *Lateral view*: Obtain periodically to determine the depth:
    ◊ Once contact is made with superior aspect of the vertebral body, advance in lateral view until needle tip is 2–3 cm past the edge of the vertebral body

- ◊ Continuously aspirate while advancing. If blood is encountered, continue to advance until aspiration stops
- ◊ Maintain osseous contact with the vertebral body wall to avoid straying too lateral.
6. Confirm placement with contrast in AP and lateral views. Contrast should be anterior to the aorta.

REFERENCE

1. Chua WH, Bogduk N. The surgical anatomy of thoracic facet denervation. Acta Neurochir (Wien). 1995;136(3-4):140-4.

Chapter 5

Pelvis, Rectum and Perineum

SUPERIOR HYPOGASTRIC PLEXUS BLOCK: POSTERIOR APPROACH

Indications
- Endometriosis, proctalgia fugax, radiation enteritis, testicular cancer pain, rectal tenesmus.
- Other genitourinary, gynecologic, colorectal, and chronic pelvic pain.

Advantages
- Injectate is intended to spread to both superior and inferior hypogastric ganglia, providing broader coverage of pain.
- It provides both diagnostic information and therapeutic benefit.
- If successful, can proceed to chemical radiofrequency ablation (RFA) for prolonged benefits.

Disadvantages/Complications
Epidural or intrathecal injection, intradiscal injection, hypotension, iliac artery/view injury/injection.

Injectate
15 mL of bupivacaine 0.25–0.5% ± 40–80 mg of methylprednisolone or steroid of choice.

Techniques
1. *Patient position:* Prone
2. *Target:* Inferior portion of the anterior L5 vertebral body (the ganglion lies at the sacral promontory point, anterior to the sacral ala).
3. *Anteroposterior (AP) view:* Square off the L5 vertebral body.
4. *Oblique view (Figs. 5.1A and B):*
   ◊ Rotate ipsilateral until tip of transverse process (TP) is aligned with the vertebral body (usually 25–35°)
   ◊ Then, tilt cephalad 20–25°. This optimizes the needle trajectory, directing the injectate inferiorly toward the ganglia.
5. Advance spinal needle (6–8 inch × 22 G) toward the inferior portion of the anterior L5 vertebral body.
6. *Lateral view:* Advance further in this view until the tip is just anterior to the vertebral body (Fig. 5.2A).

Chapter 5: Pelvis, Rectum and Perineum

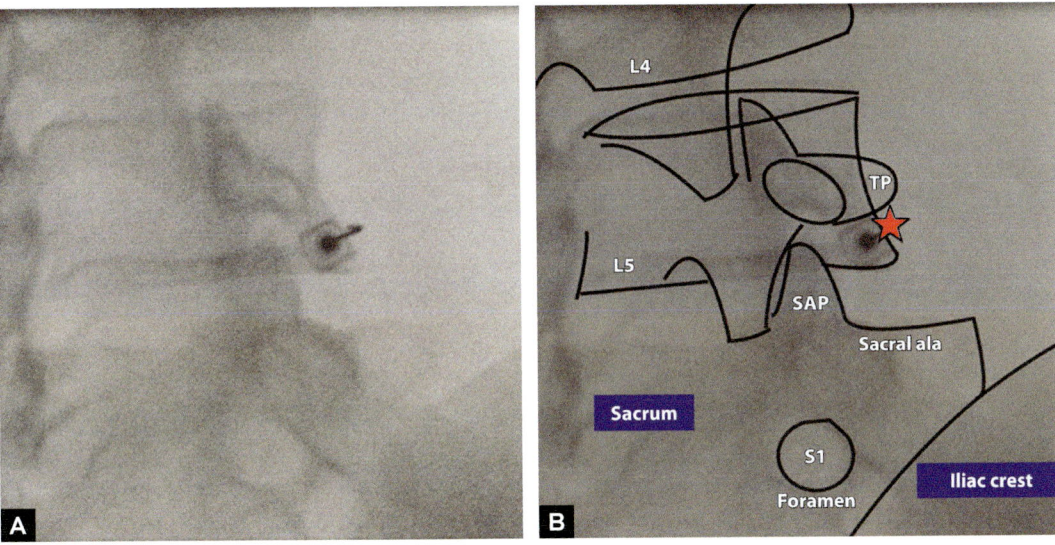

Figs. 5.1A and B: Superior hypogastric plexus block. (A) Ipsilateral rotation of 25–35° and a 20–25° cephalad tilt; (B) Ipsilateral rotation of 25–35° and a 20–25° cephalad tilt (labeled).
(TP: Transverse process; SAP: Superior articular process).

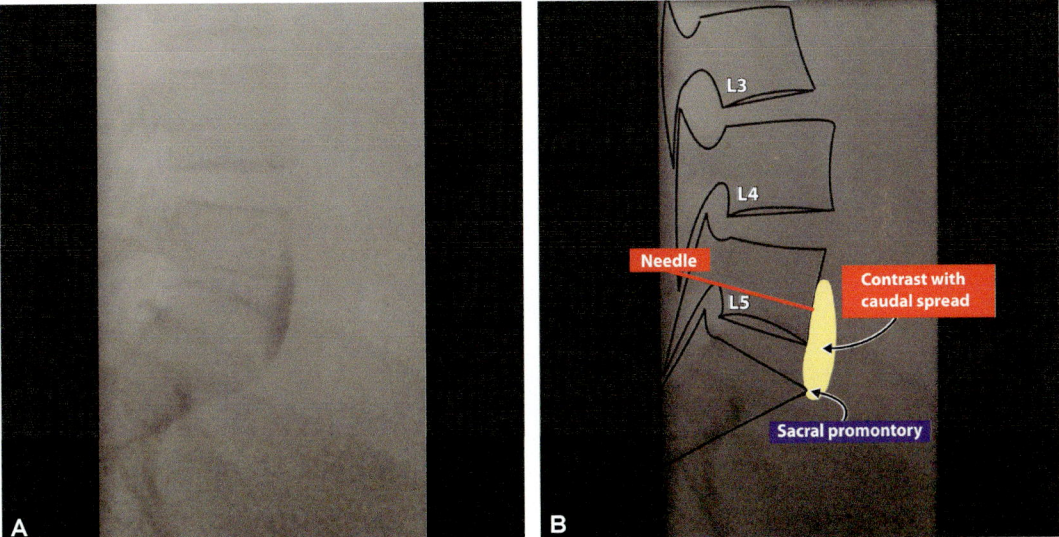

Figs. 5.2A and B: Superior hypogastric plexus block—lateral view. (A) Contrast spread anterior to the vertebral body and down toward the sacral promontory point of the sacrum; (B) Contrast spread anterior to the vertebral body (labeled).

7. Confirm placement with contrast in lateral view. The spread should be anterior to the vertebral body (Fig. 5.2B).
8. Confirm placement with contrast in anteroposterior (AP) view. If spread does not cross midline, a bilateral injection is recommended (Figs. 5.3A and B).

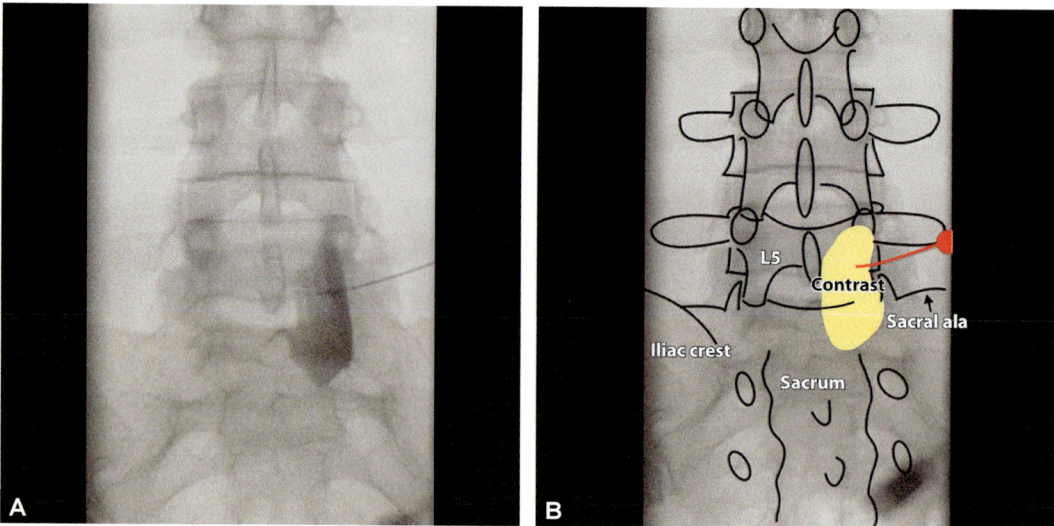

Figs. 5.3A and B: Superior hypogastric plexus block—anteroposterior (AP) view. (A) Contrast spread; (B) Contrast spread (labeled).

GANGLION IMPAR BLOCK:
SACROCOCCYGEAL/INTERCOCCYGEAL JOINT APPROACH

Indications
- Treatment of sympathetically mediated pain in the rectum and perineal region.
- Pain secondary to malignancy (e.g. prostate, cervical, and colon cancers).
- Neuropathic pain.
- Postsurgical pain in the pelvic, genital, rectal, and perineal regions.
- Controversial treatment for coccydynia (alternatively may block the bilateral S5 and coccygeal nerve).

Advantage
Neurolysis using phenol or other chemoneurolytic substance versus "pulsed" RFA of the ganglion impar can provide longer-lasting pain relief.

Disadvantages/Complications
- Higher risk for infection given location and close proximity to pelvic viscera.
- Bowel perforation.
- Epidural spread.

Injectate
5 mL of bupivacaine 0.5% ± 40 mg methylprednisolone or steroid of choice.

Techniques
1. *Patient position:* Prone
2. *Target:* Sacrococcygeal or intercoccygeal joints.

3. *Anteroposterior view (Figs. 5.4A and B):* Identify the coccyx, the sacrococcygeal joint, and mark midline.
   ◊ *Optimize view:* Caudal tilt of 5–10° to better visualize the coccyx.
4. *Lateral view:* Start procedure in this view (Figs. 5.5A and B).
5. Advance spinal needle (1–3.5 inch × 25 G) through the target joint until the tip is resting just anterior to the coccyx and posterior to the rectum.

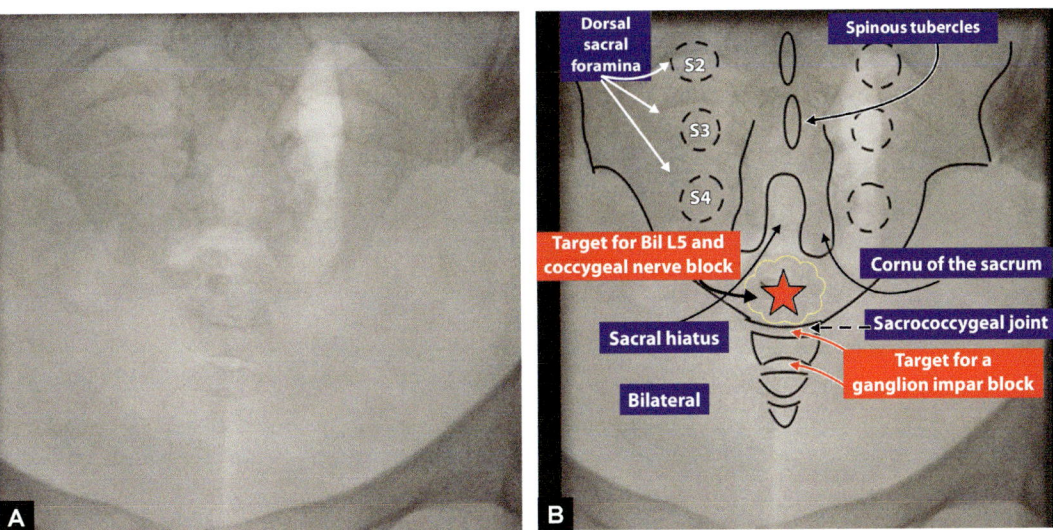

Figs. 5.4A and B: (A) Ganglion impar block—anteroposterior (AP) view. (A) A caudal tilt of 5–10° to identify midline and the sacrococcygeal joint; (B) A caudal tilt of 5–10° to identify midline and the sacrococcygeal joint (labeled).

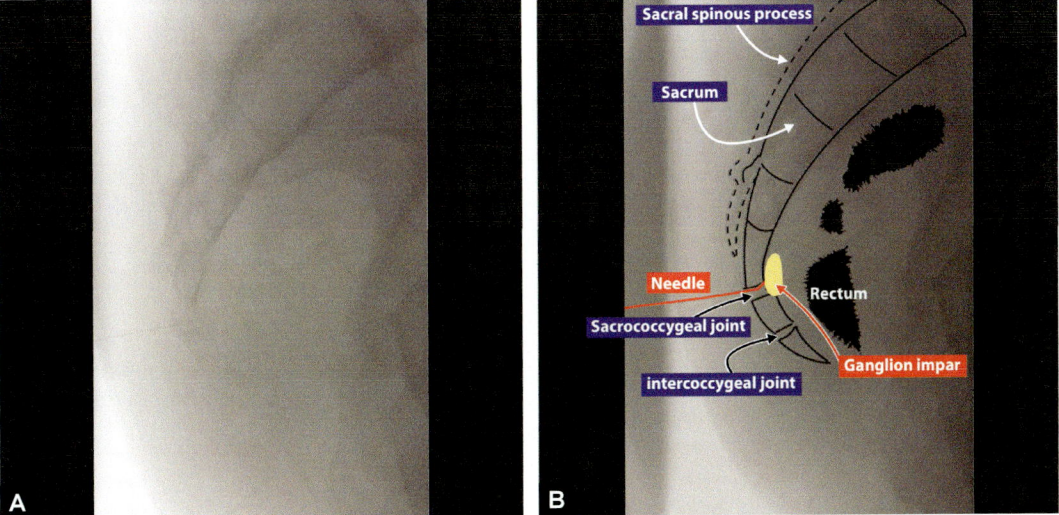

Figs. 5.5A and B: Ganglion impar block—lateral view. (A) The needle is advanced through the sacrococcygeal joint until the tip of the needle is just anterior to the joint; (B) Contrast spread (labeled).

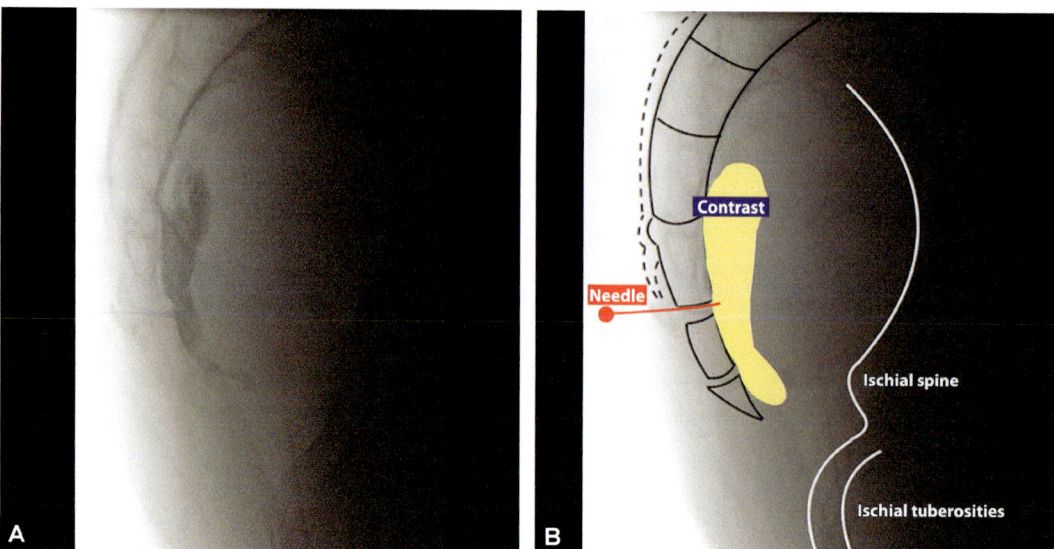

Figs. 5.6A and B: Ganglion impar block—lateral view. (A) Contrast spread along the curvature of the sacrum and coccyx; (B) Contrast spread (labeled).

6. Confirm placement with contrast in AP and lateral views (flow should be bilateral) (Figs. 5.6A and B).
7. Vascular uptake is frequently seen so needle tip should be adjusted to avoid vasculature.

PUDENDAL NERVE BLOCK
Indication
Pain in the anal region, perineum, scrotum, penis or vulva.

Advantages
- Diagnostic and therapeutic intervention.
- If successful, it can proceed to pulsed RFA.

Disadvantages/Complications
- There are both motor and sensory components and therefore, traditional RFA cannot be performed.
- Risk of bowel and bladder incontinence if a bilateral injection is performed.
- Neurovascular injection.
- Sciatic nerve block.

Injectate
3-4 mL of bupivacaine 0.5% ± 20 mg of methylprednisolone or steroid of choice per side.

Techniques
1. *Patient position:* Prone
2. *Target:* Just lateral to the tip of the ischial spine.
3. *Anteroposterior view (Figs. 5.7A and B):* Identify acetabulum and femoral head.
    ◊ Tilt caudal 5-10° and rotate ipsilateral 5-10°. This brings the ischial spine into view.

Chapter 5: Pelvis, Rectum and Perineum

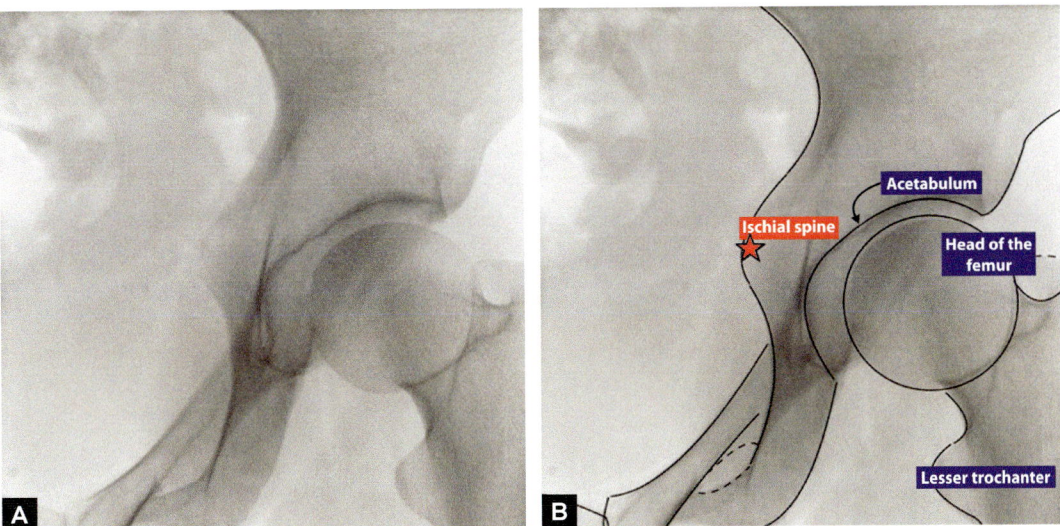

Figs. 5.7A and B: Pudendal nerve block—identify the femoral head on an anteroposterior (AP) view. (A) The rotate ipsilateral 5–10° with a 5–10° caudal tilt. This helps bring out the ischial spine; (B) 5–10° ipsilateral rotation with a 5–10° caudal tilt (labeled).

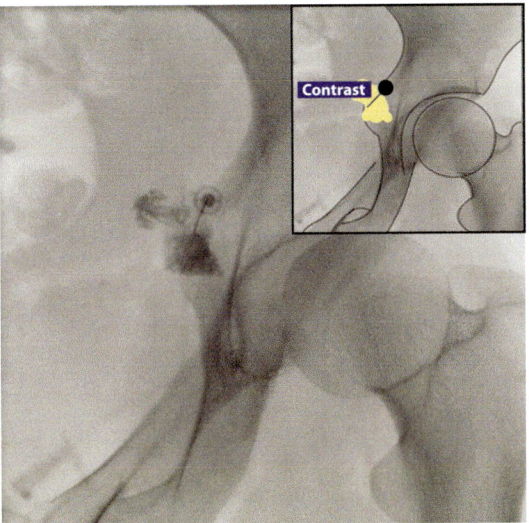

Fig. 5.8: Pudendal nerve block—contrast spread.

4. Advance spinal needle (3.5 inch × 22–25 G) toward the medial edge of the target until osseous contact is made.
5. Confirm placement with contrast (Fig. 5.8).

Chapter 6

Lumbar Spine, Hips and Lower Extremities

LUMBAR INTERLAMINAR EPIDURAL STEROID INJECTION: PARASAGITTAL APPROACH

Indication
- Lumbar radiculopathy.
- Lumbar spinal stenosis.

Advantage
Useful in treating multilevel pathology or bilateral symptoms.

Disadvantages/Complications
- *Standard epidural steroid injection (ESI) risks*: Unintended dural puncture with postdural puncture headache (PDPH), infection, hematomas, nerve injury, spinal cord infarct, worsening pain, etc.
- Intradiscal injection/entry

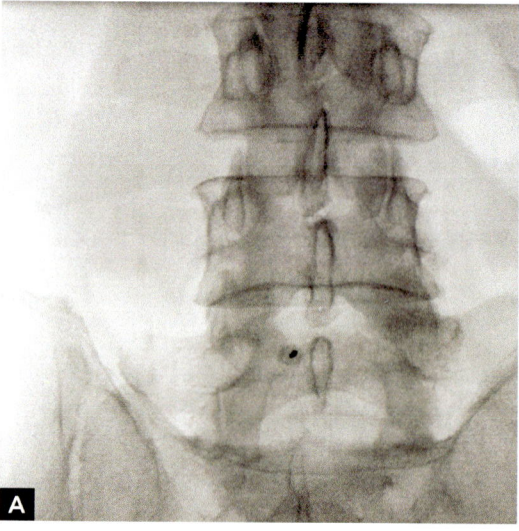 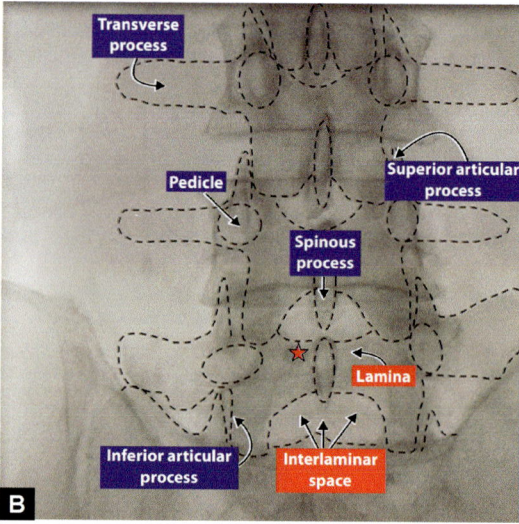

Figs. 6.1A and B: (A) Lumbar interlaminar epidural steroid injection (ESI)—anteroposterior (AP) view. Caudal or cephalad tilt depending on the degree of lordosis of the spine. Above L4/L5 may require a 5–10° caudal tilt to "open" the interspace; (B) Lumbar interlaminar ESI—AP view (labeled).

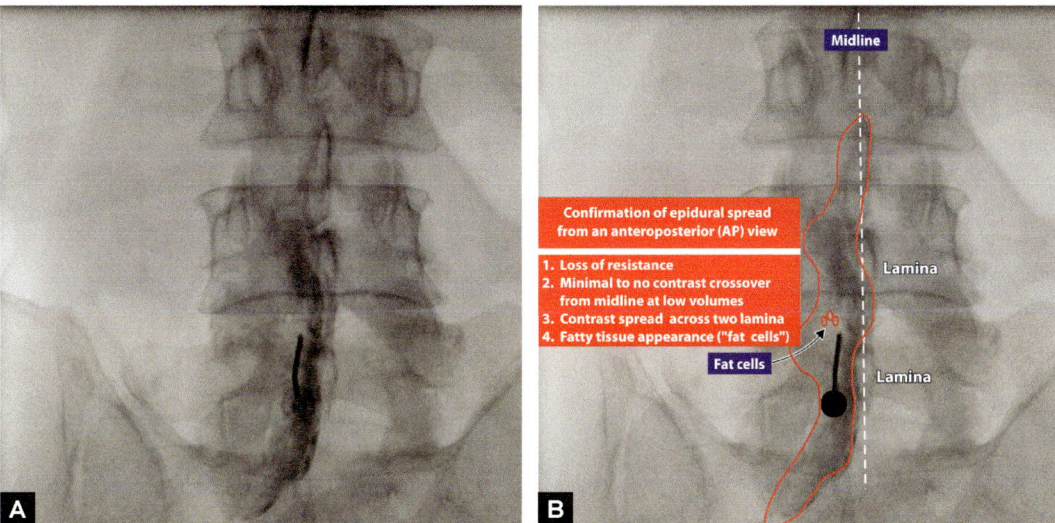

Figs. 6.2A and B: Lumbar interlaminar ESI—AP view. (A) Contrast spread; (B) Confirmation of epidural spread (labeled).

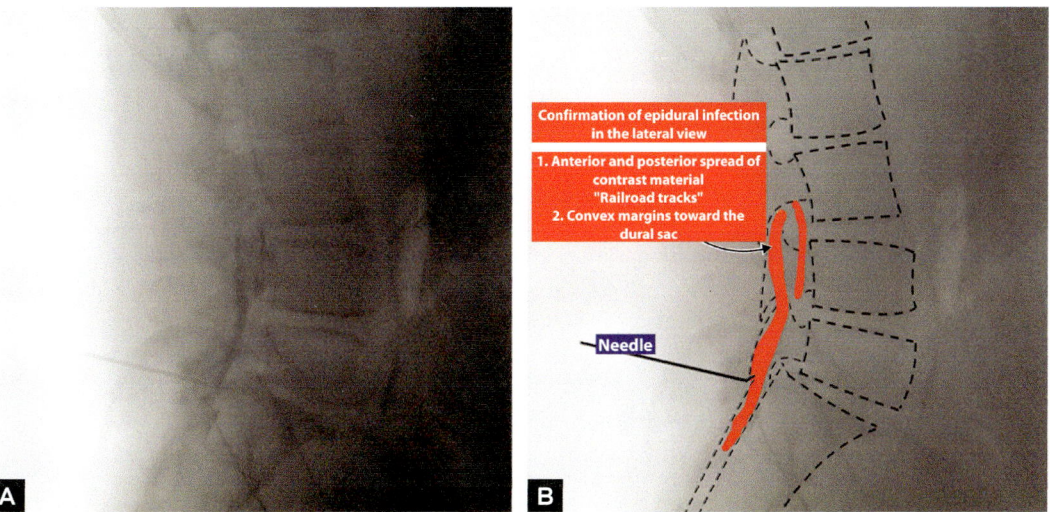

Figs. 6.3A and B: Lumbar interlaminar ESI—lateral view. (A) Contrast spread; (B) Confirmation of epidural spread (labeled).

Injectate

40–80 mg of methylprednisolone or steroid of choice + 1 mL preservative-free normal saline (PFNS) + 1 mL bupivacaine 0.25–0.5%.

Techniques

1. *Patient position*: Prone.
2. *Target*: Interspace just lateral to midline on the symptomatic side.

3. *anteroposterior (AP) view*: Square off vertebral body at the level of the injection or until the interspace is maximally opened (5–15° caudate vs cephalad tilt) (Figs. 6.1A and B).
4. Advance Tuohy needle (3.5–6 inch × 18–20G) toward the superior portion of the lamina at the respective interspace (i.e. L4/L5 interspace—contact the superior portion of the L5 lamina) just lateral to midline on the symptomatic side.
5. Once lamina is contacted, step off superiorly 2–3 mm.
    ◊ If symptoms are bilateral, direct the needle toward the middle of the interspace
    ◊ If symptoms are unilateral, angle the needle toward the symptomatic side.
6. Connect the loss of resistance (LOR) syringe to your needle and advance until loss.
7. Confirm placement with contrast in AP (Figs. 6.2A and B) and lateral views (Figs. 6.3A and B).

LUMBAR TRANSFORAMINAL EPIDURAL STEROID INJECTION: SUBPEDICULAR APPROACH

Indications
- Lumbar radiculopathy.
- Manage symptoms of lumbar spinal stenosis.

Advantages
- Targets a specific nerve root.
- Needle tip bound within the "safe triangle" (superiorly by the inferior border superior pedicle, laterally by an imaginary line between the lateral edges of the pedicles, and medially by the spinal nerve root).
- Injectate is placed "closer" to the site of neural impingement (vs other transforaminal approaches).

Disadvantages/Complications
- Intravascular—higher likelihood of a medullary artery injection compared to other lumbar transforaminal ESI (TFESI) techniques (highest at L2 and lowest at the L4 level).[1]
- Unable to use this approach when superior articular process (SAP) or osteophytes obstruct the target.
- *Standard ESI risks*: Infection, hematomas, nerve injury, spinal cord infarct, worsening pain, etc.
- Inadvertent facet injection

Injectate
4–8 mg of dexamethasone or steroid of choice (nonparticulate preferred) + 1 mL PFNS + 1 mL of bupivacaine 0.25–0.5%.

Techniques
1. *Patient position*: Prone.
2. *Target*: 6 o'clock position of the pedicle, just posterior to the vertebral body.
3. *Anteroposterior view*:
    ◊ If the lamina obscures the target, rotate ipsilateral 5–10°
    ◊ If the transverse process (TP) obscures the target, tilt caudal 5–10° (Figs. 6.4A and B).

4. Advance the spinal needle (3.5–6 inch × 22–25 G) coaxial to the 6 o'clock position of the pedicle. Target region is within the foramen just posterior the vertebral body (Fig. 6.4A).
5. *Lateral view*: Use intermittently to determine depth and location within the foramen (Figs. 6.5A and B).
6. Confirm placement with contrast under live fluoroscopy in AP (Fig. 6.6) and lateral views.

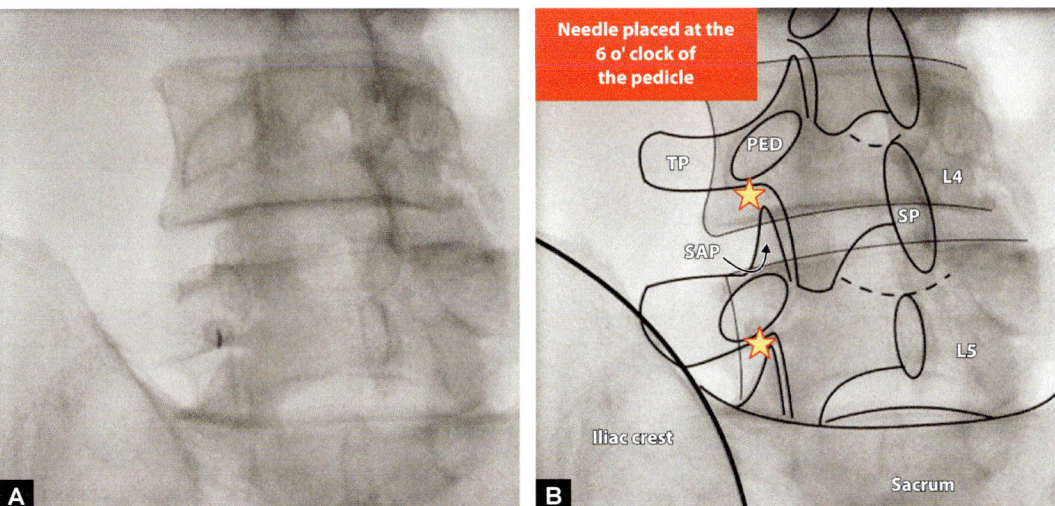

Figs. 6.4A and B: (A) Lumbar transforaminal epidural steroid injection (TFESI): subpedicular approach—AP view. Optional 5–10° ipsilateral rotation with a 5–10° caudal tilt to optimize view. Target the 6 o'clock position of the pedicle; (B) Lumbar TFESI: subpedicular approach—AP view (labeled).

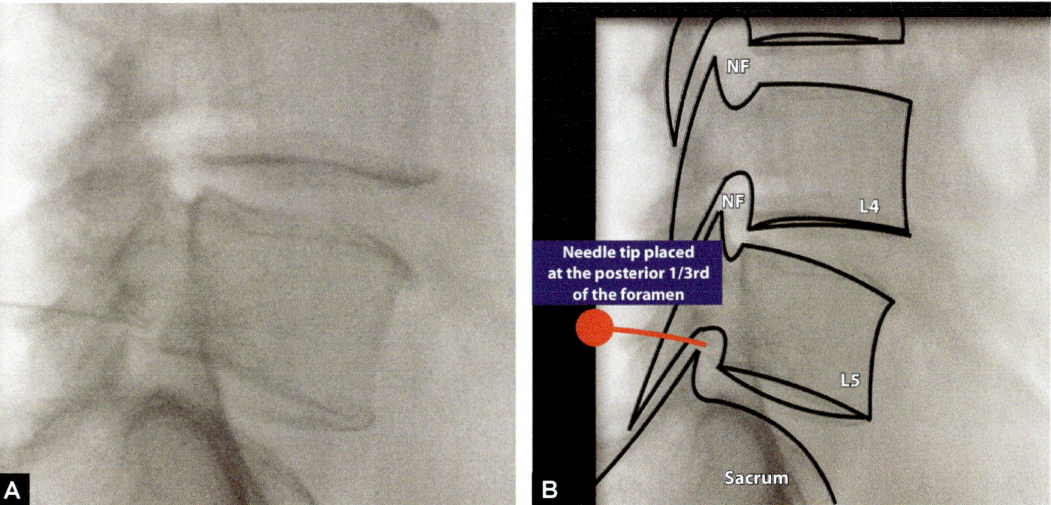

Figs. 6.5A and B: (A) Lumbar TFESI: subpedicular approach—lateral view. Needle placed at the posterior one-third of the foramen; (B) Lumbar TFESI: subpedicular approach—lateral view (labeled).

LUMBAR TRANSFORAMINAL EPIDURAL STEROID INJECTION: SUPRANEURAL APPROACH

Indications
- Lumbar radiculopathy.
- Lumbar spinal stenosis.

Advantages
- Avoids contacting the floor of the intervertebral foramen, where radicular arteries potentially lie, therefore possibly reducing the risk of intra-arterial injection.[1]
- Needle tip bound within the "safe triangle" (superiorly by the inferior border superior pedicle, laterally by an imaginary line between the lateral edges of the pedicles, and medially by the spinal nerve root). Theoretically avoids injuring nerve root.

Disadvantage/Complication
Standard ESI risks: Infection, hematomas, nerve injury, spinal cord infarct, worsening pain, etc.

Injectate
4–8 mg of dexamethasone or the steroid of choice (nonparticulate preferred) + 1 mL PFNS + 1 mL of bupivacaine 0.25–0.5%.

Techniques
1. *Patient position*: Prone.
2. *Target*: 6 o'clock position of pedicle at mid to posterior one-third of foramen.
3. *Anteroposterior view*: Square off vertebral body at level of the injection.
4. *Oblique view*: Rotate ipsilateral 15–20° or until the lamina has been medially rotated off the pedicle (Figs. 6.7A and B).

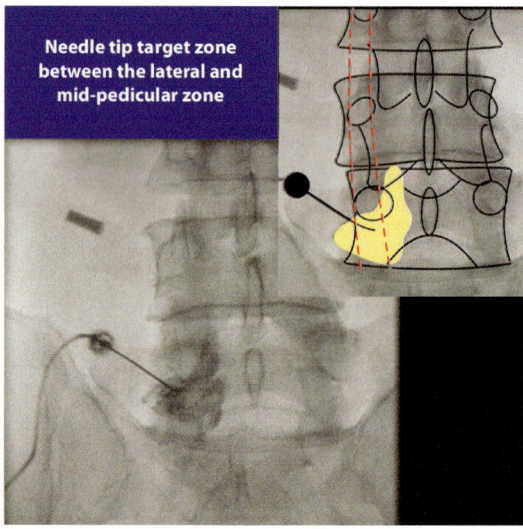

Fig. 6.6: Lumbar TFESI: subpedicular approach—AP view. Contrast spread.

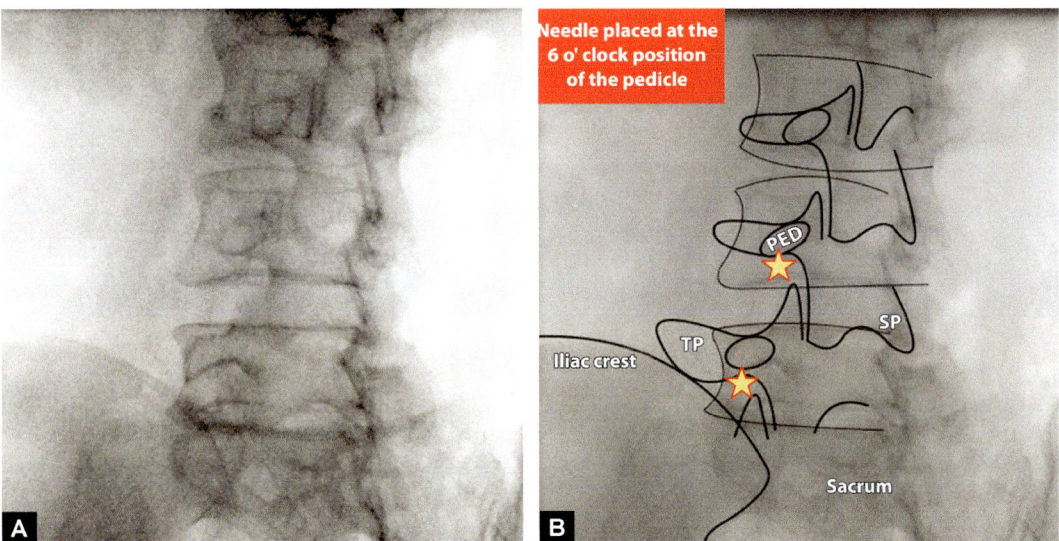

Figs. 6.7A and B: (A) Lumbar TFESI: supraneural approach—ipsilateral rotation 15–20°; (B) Lumbar TFESI: supraneural approach—ipsilateral rotation 15–20° (labeled).

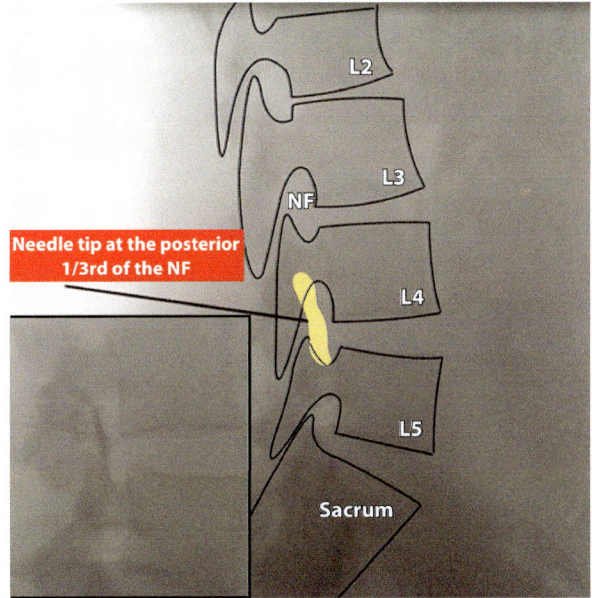

Fig. 6.8: Lumbar TFESI: supraneural approach—lateral view. Contrast spread.

5. Advance spinal needle (3.5–6 inch × 22–25G) toward target.
6. *Lateral view*: Confirm appropriate depth of needle tip.
7. Confirm placement with contrast under live fluoroscopy in AP and lateral views (Fig. 6.8).

LUMBAR TRANSFORAMINAL EPIDURAL STEROID INJECTION: RETRONEURAL APPROACH

Indications
- Lumbar radiculopathy.
- Lumbar spinal stenosis.

Advantages
- Useful when the targeted nerve is displaced upward by a disk herniation or foraminal stenosis, rendering "safe triangle" unsafe in avoiding nerve contact.
- Useful when SAP or osteophytes obstruct a subpedicular technique.
- Possibly lower risk of intra-arterial injection compared to the subpedicular or supraneural approaches.[1]
- By walking off lamina, provides security of a bony landmark and a sense of depth.

Disadvantage/Complication
Standard ESI risks: Infection, hematomas, nerve injury, spinal cord infarct, worsening pain, etc.

Injectate
4–8 mg of dexamethasone or steroid of choice (nonparticulate preferred) + 1 mL PFNS + 1 mL of bupivacaine 0.25–0.5%.

Techniques
1. *Patient position*: Prone.
2. *Target*: Just lateral to lamina and inferior to TP.
3. *Anteroposterior view*: May rotate ipsilateral 5–10° until lamina edge bisects pedicle (Figs. 6.9A and B).
   ◊ If the SAP obstructs the target zone, tilt caudal 5–10°.

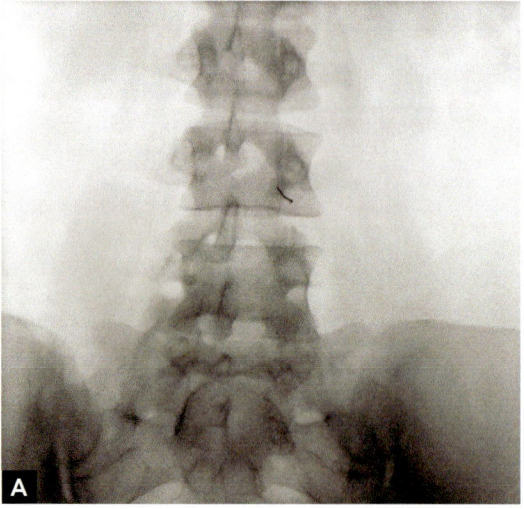 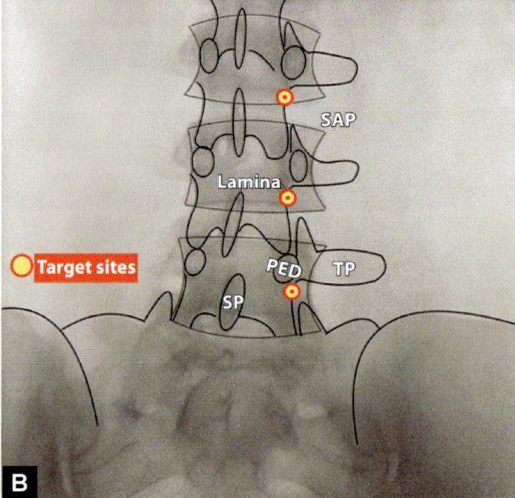

Figs. 6.9A and B: (A) Lumbar TFESI: retroneural approach—AP view. Optional: ipsilateral rotation 5° or until the lamina bisects the pedicle; (B) Lumbar TFESI: retroneural approach—AP view (labeled).

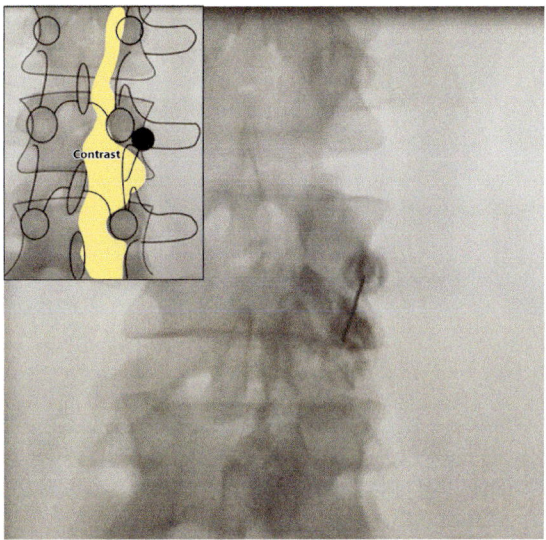

Fig. 6.10: Lumbar TFESI: retroneural approach—AP view. Contrast spread.

4. Advance spinal needle (3.6–6 inch × 22–25 G) until tip contacts edge of the lamina.
5. Then walk off 2–3 mm inferior to the TP.
6. *Lateral view*: To determine depth and location within the foramen (tip should be at the posterior one-third of the foramen).
7. Confirm placement with contrast under live fluoroscopy in AP (Fig. 6.10) and lateral views.

LUMBAR TRANSFORAMINAL EPIDURAL STEROID INJECTION: INFRANEURAL APPROACH (KAMBIN'S TRIANGLE)

Indications
- Lumbar radiculopathy.
- Lumbar spinal stenosis.

Advantages
- Avoids contacting the spinal nerve and artery (nerve and artery traditionally lie inferior to the pedicle and superior to the SAP and respective disk).
- By walking off the inferior SAP, provides a sense of depth and potentially avoids the need for a confirmatory lateral view.
- Theoretically least likely to result in paresthesia, nerve injury, or intravascular injection when compared to other transforaminal approaches.

Disadvantages/Complications
- Highest risk for intradiskal injection.
- *Standard ESI risks*: Infection, hematomas, nerve injury, spinal cord infarct, worsening pain, etc.

Injectate

4–8 mg of dexamethasone or steroid of choice (nonparticulate preferred) + 1 mL PFNS + 1 mL of bupivacaine 0.25–0.5%.

Techniques

1. *Patient position*: Prone.
2. *Target*: Just lateral to the upper two-thirds of the SAP.
3. *Anteroposterior view*: Square off the vertebral body at the level of the injection.
4. *Oblique view (Figs. 6.11 and 6.12)*:
   ◊ Rotate ipsilateral at least 30° or until the SAP sits across one-third to one-half of the respective disk. This trajectory facilitates walking posteromedial off the SAP and into the epidural space
   ◊ If the entire SAP overlies disk only, tilt caudal until superior aspect of SAP lies over vertebral body. This is done to avoid intradiskal injection should the needle tip stray deeper than intended.
5. Advance spinal needle (3.5–6 inch × 22–25G) toward the upper portion of the SAP.
6. Then walk off 1–2 mm and redirect medially.
7. *Anteroposterior view*: Advance needle medially until the tip of the needle lies at or just lateral to the facet or zygapophyseal joint.
8. Confirm placement with contrast under live fluoroscopy (Figs. 6.13A and B).

CAUDAL EPIDURAL STEROID INJECTION

Indications

Lumbar radiculopathy with or without axial back pain.
- Postlaminectomy syndrome.
- Severe lumbar stenosis where safe interlaminar or transforaminal access may be difficult.

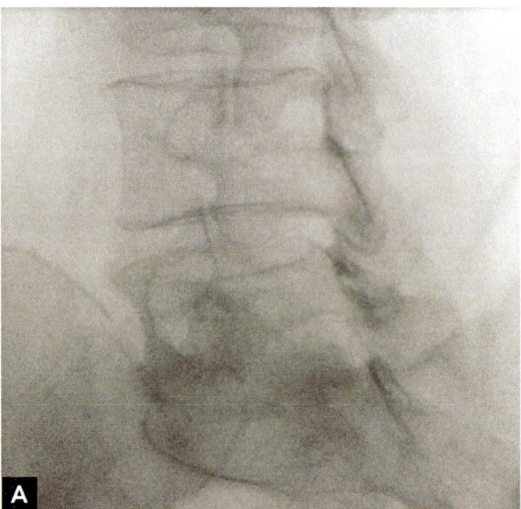
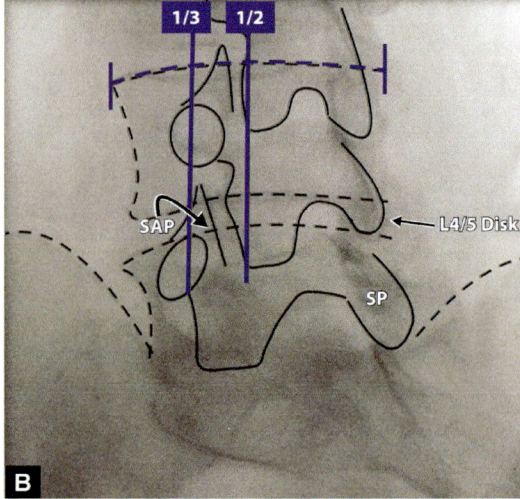

Figs. 6.11A and B: (A) Lumbar TFESI: infraneural approach—25–35° ipsilateral rotation; (B) Lumbar TFESI: infraneural approach—25–35° ipsilateral rotation or until the superior articular process (SAP) is between one-third to one-half the diameter of the respective vertebral body (labeled).

Chapter 6: Lumbar Spine, Hips and Lower Extremities

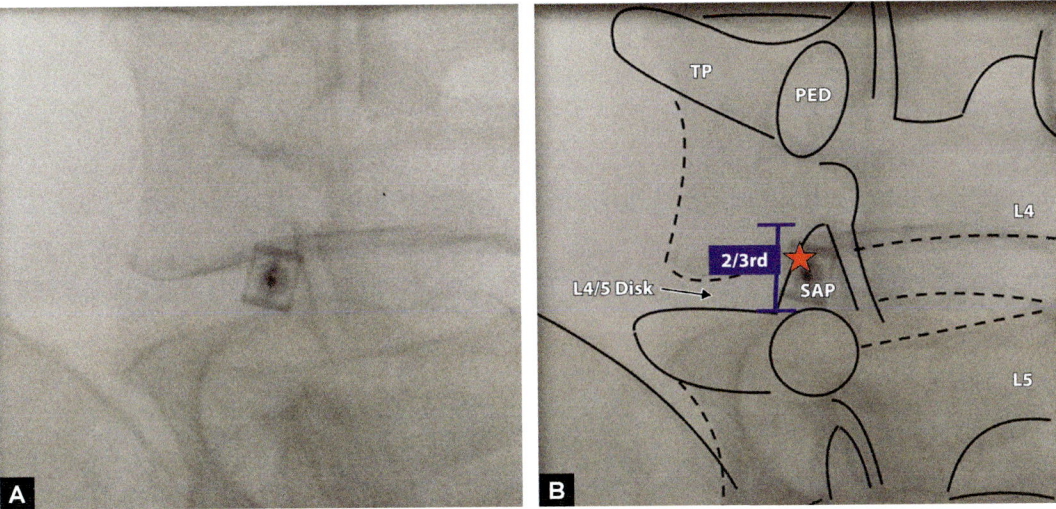

Figs. 6.12A and B: (A) Lumbar TFESI: infraneural approach—25–35° ipsilateral rotation (magnified); (B) Lumbar TFESI: infraneural approach—25–35° ipsilateral rotation (labeled).

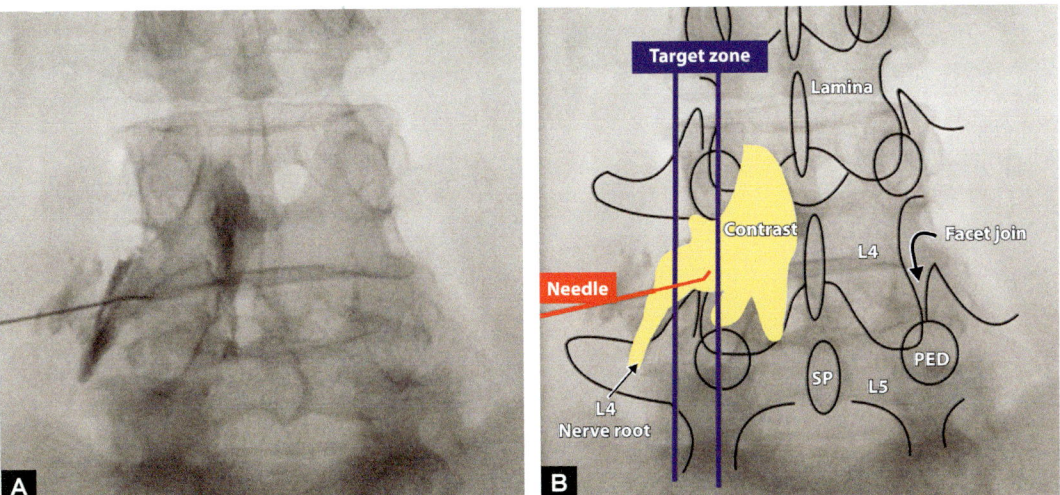

Figs. 6.13A and B: (A) Lumbar TFESI: infraneural approach—AP view. Contrast spread; (B) Lumbar TFESI: infraneural approach: AP view. Contrast spread (labeled).

Advantages
- Useful when difficult lumbar visualization or difficult access is encountered (i.e. hardware or postsurgical changes).
- Allows catheter placement for flexibility in neural targeting.

Disadvantages/Complications
- Nonselective high volume block.
- Unreliable spread of local anesthetic.

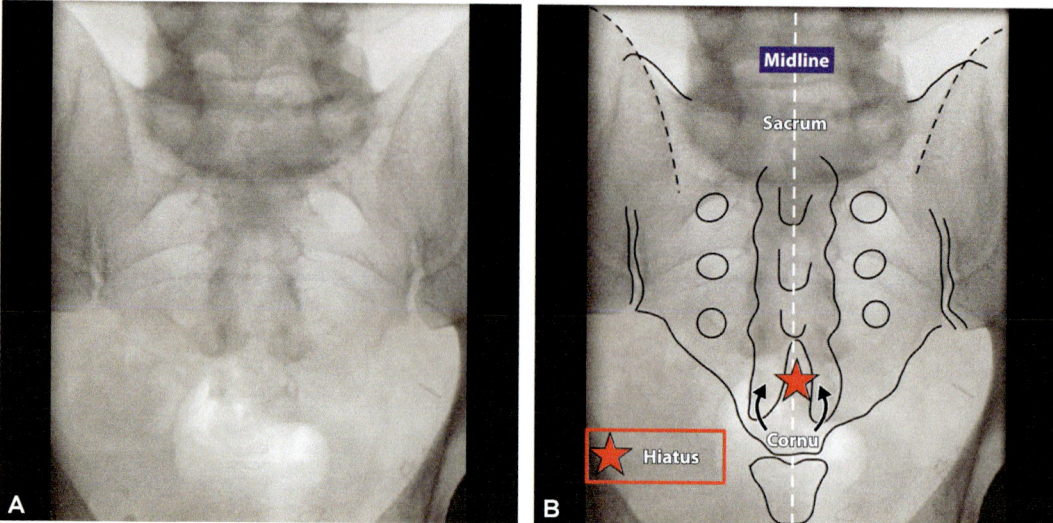

Figs. 6.14A and B: (A) Caudal ESI—AP view. Identify midline and the sacral hiatus; (B) Caudal ESI—AP view (labeled).

- Limited to the lower lumbar and sacral nerve roots.
- Risk of intrathecal access/injection with catheter tip (thecal sac terminates at S2).

Injectate
Total 5–25 mL (10 mL to reach L5, 15 mL for L4).
- 40–80 mg of methylprednisolone (or steroid of choice) + 2–3 mL of bupivacaine 0.5% diluted in PFNS.
- Without catheter: dilution of anesthetic is necessary to prevent dense sacral block.

Techniques
1. *Patient position*: Prone.
2. *Target*: Sacral hiatus.
3. *Anteroposterior view*: Palpate and mark the sacral cornu and hiatus, mark midline (Figs. 6.14A and B).
4. *Lateral view*: Identify the sacral hiatus (bordered by the sacral cornu) (Figs. 6.15A and B).
5. Advance spinal needle (3.5 inch × 22G or 25G), at a 45° angle through the sacral hiatus toward the S3 foramen.
6. Confirm placement with contrast in AP and lateral views (where a "Christmas tree" appearance should be noted with adequate volume) (Figs. 6.16A and B).
7. *Optional*: A catheter can be placed using an 18G or 16G epidural introducer needle with a 19G or 21G "Racz catheter", respectively.

LUMBAR INTRA-ARTICULAR FACET JOINT INJECTION
Indications
- Lumbar spondylosis.
- Axial back pain without radicular symptoms.

Chapter 6: Lumbar Spine, Hips and Lower Extremities

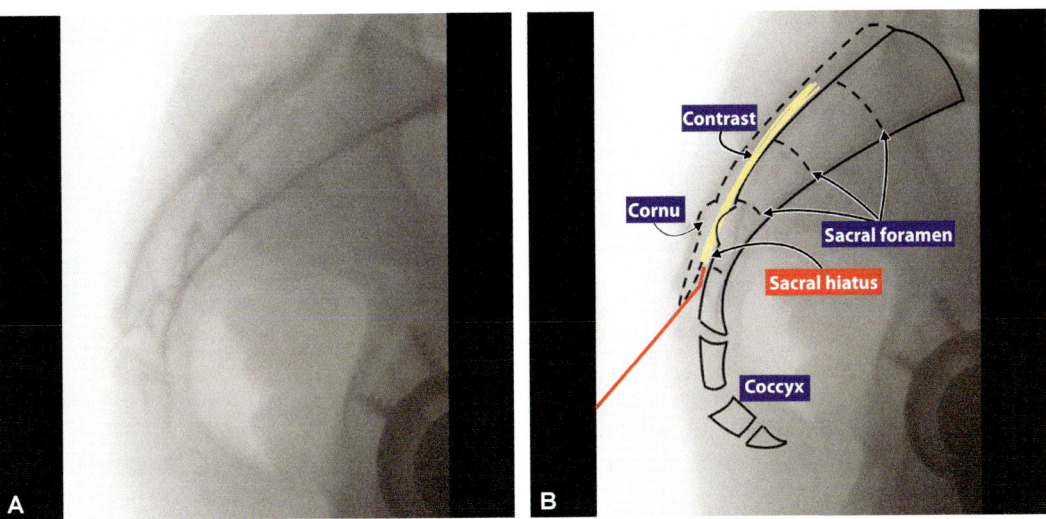

Figs. 6.15A and B: (A) Caudal ESI—lateral view; (B) Caudal ESI—lateral view with contrast (labeled).

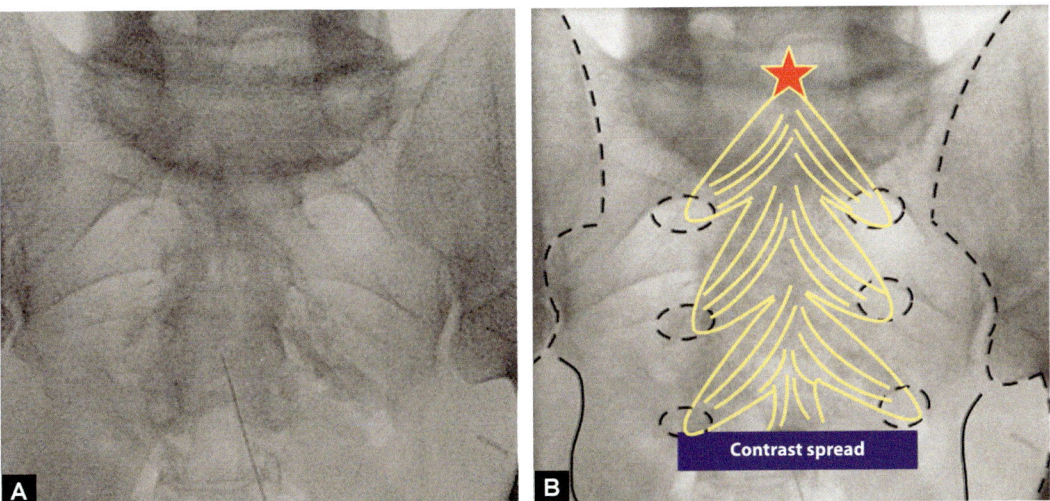

Figs. 6.16A and B: (A) Caudal ESI—AP view with contrast. "Christmas tree" appearance of contrast; (B) Caudal ESI—AP view with contrast.

Advantages
- Intra-articular injections are diagnostic and therapeutic interventions.
- With enough volume, injectate can also achieve epidural spread and indirectly provide similar benefits to an ESI.

Disadvantages/Complications
- Exacerbation of pain.
- Risk of epidural spread if greater than 1.5 mL of volume is injected into the facet joint.

Injectate

0.5–1 mL of 40–80 mg of methylprednisolone or steroid of choice + bupivacaine 0.5% divided among the joints to be injected.

Techniques

1. *Patient position*: Prone.
2. *Target*: Superior or inferior portion of the facet joint.
3. *Anteroposterior view*: Square off vertebral body at the level of the injection.
4. *Oblique view*: Rotate ipsilateral until the joint lines are clearly visible (usually 25–35°) (Figs. 6.17A and B).
5. Advance spinal needle (3.5–6 inch × 22–25G) toward the superior portion of the facet joint (Figs. 6.18A and B).
   ◊ *Tip*: Since facet joints have a "C" shape contour, edging toward the medial border of the facet joint and redirecting slightly laterally may assist with placement.
6. Confirm placement with a small amount of contrast (the joint can hold a little more than 1 mL of volume).

LUMBAR MEDIAL BRANCH BLOCK AND RADIOFREQUENCY ABLATION

Indications

- Lumbar spondylosis.
- Facet arthrosis.
- Axial back pain without radicular symptoms.

Advantages

- Medial branch block (MBB) provides diagnostic information.
- Chemoneurolytic ablation can be easily done using the MBB technique and by administering a chemoneurolytic substance (phenol, methylene blue, 50% dextrose).
- Radiofrequency ablation (RFA) provides longer-lasting relief.

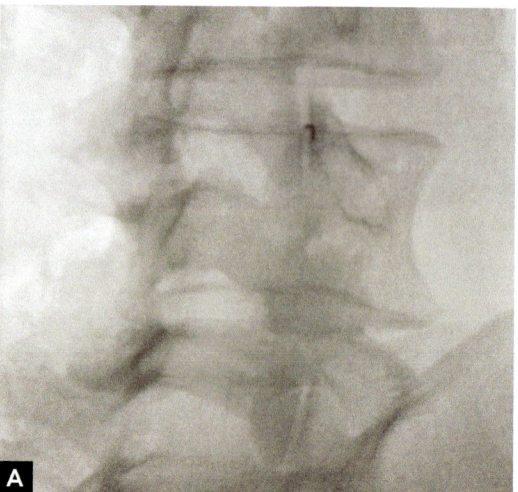 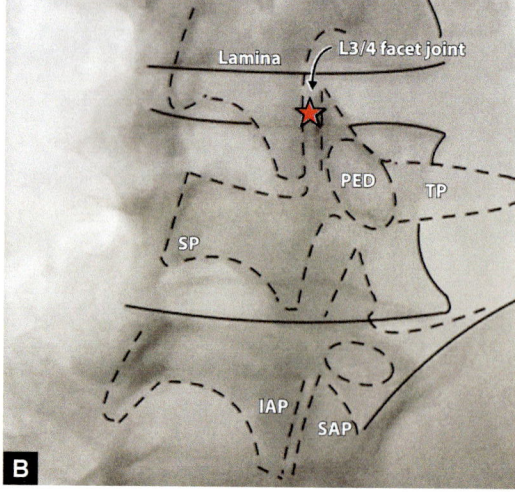

Figs. 6.17A and B: (A) Lumbar facet Intra-articular injection. 25–35° ipsilateral rotation or until the facet joint lines appear as train tracks; (B) Lumbar facet intra-articular injection. 25–35° ipsilateral rotation (labeled).

Chapter 6: Lumbar Spine, Hips and Lower Extremities

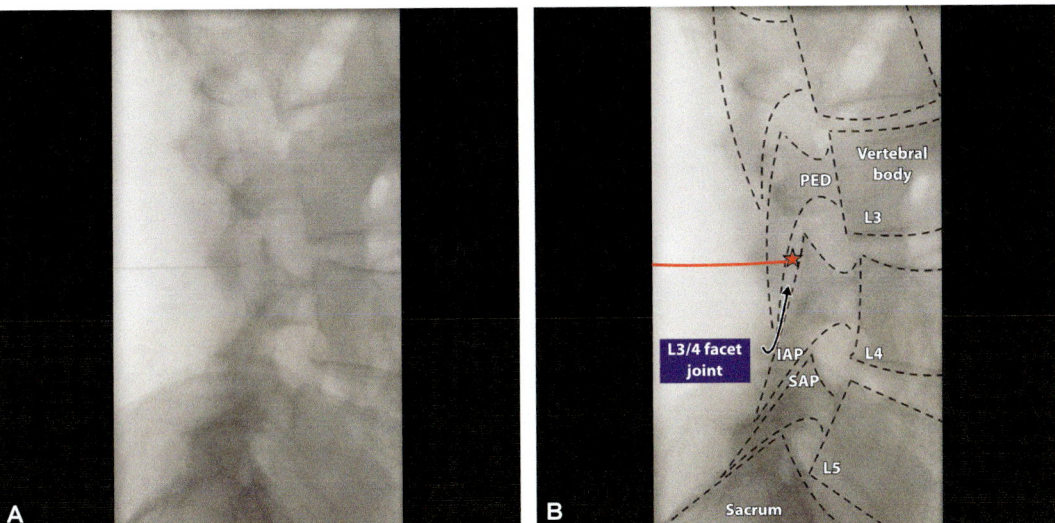

Figs. 6.18A and B: (A) Lateral view. Lumbar facet intra-articular injection. Needle placed at the midpoint of the facet joint; (B) Lateral view. Lumbar facet intra-articular injection (labeled).

Disadvantages/Complications
- Diagnostic blocks provide short-term duration (<12 hours if only bupivacaine is used).
- Minimal sedatives can falsify diagnostic information (i.e. giving midazolam causes muscle relaxation, and fentanyl can diminish pain scores).
- Requires multiple levels of injections as each joint is innervated by the medial branch at the level and the level above the joint (i.e. L4-L5 joint by L3 MB and L4 MB).

Injectate
- Medial branch block: 0.5 mL of bupivacaine 0.5% at each level.
- Chemoneurolysis: 1 mL 50% dextrose or substance of choice.
- Radiofrequency ablation: Once complete, administer 1 mL bupivacaine 0.5% with or without 1 mL steroid of choice divided among all the levels.

Techniques
1. *Patient position*: Prone.
2. *Anteroposterior view*: Square off vertebral body at the level of the injection.
3. *Target*: Junction of the SAP and TP [or ala for L5 dorsal ramus (DR)].
4. *Oblique view (Figs. 6.19A and B)*:
   ◊ For L1-L4 MBB: rotate ipsilateral 15–20° and tilt caudal or cranially 10–15° for clearer visualization of SAP and TP junction.
   ◊ For L1-L4 RFA: rotate ipsilateral 15–20° and tilt caudal 15–20° to facilitate needle laying across the groove of the junction.
   ◊ For L5 DR MBB or RFA: rotate ipsilateral 5–10° and tilt caudal 5–10°.
5. Advance spinal needle (3.5–6 inch × 22–25G) to the target junction. This correlates to approximately 11 o'clock (left) or 1 o'clock (right) on the pedicle (Figs. 6.20A and B).

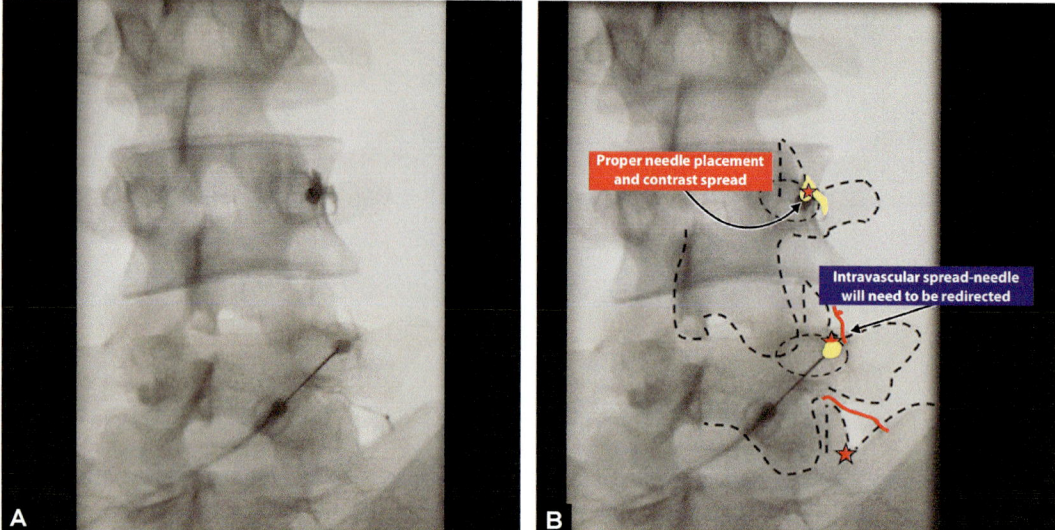

Figs. 6.19A and B: (A) Lumbar medial branch block—ipsilateral and cranial or caudal tilt of 15–20°. Of note, there is vascular uptake at the L4 medial branch site; (B) Lumbar medial branch block—oblique view.

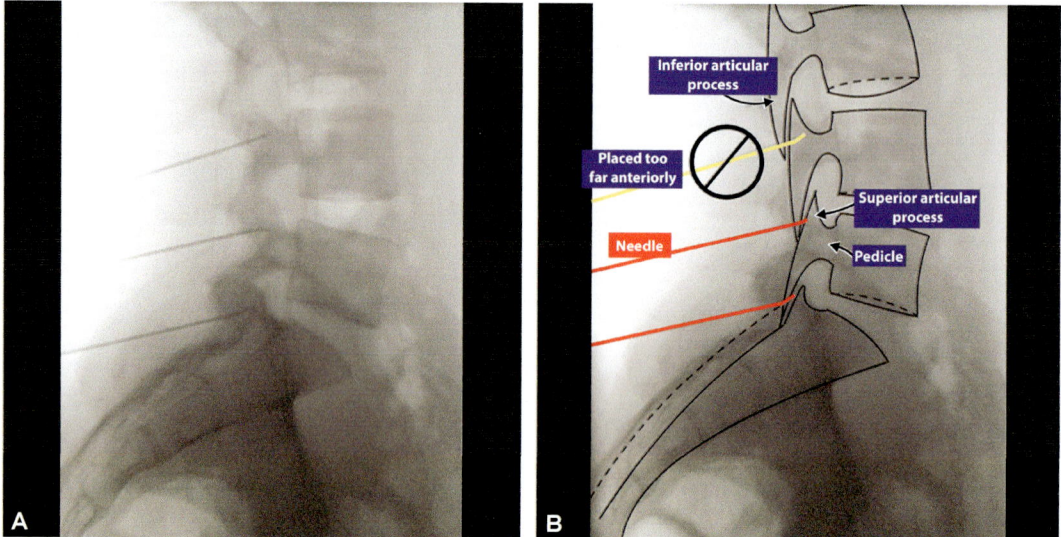

Figs. 6.20A and B: (A) Lumbar medial branch block—lateral view; (B) Lumbar medial branch block—lateral view. The needle tip should lie at the midpoint of the respective facet joint.

6. For MBB, confirm placement with a small amount of contrast and administer injectate (Figs. 6.21A and B).
7. For RFA, confirm in *lateral view* that needle is at respective joint line. Before the ablation is carried out, sensory and motor stimulation confirms there is nerve root stimulation.

Chapter 6: Lumbar Spine, Hips and Lower Extremities

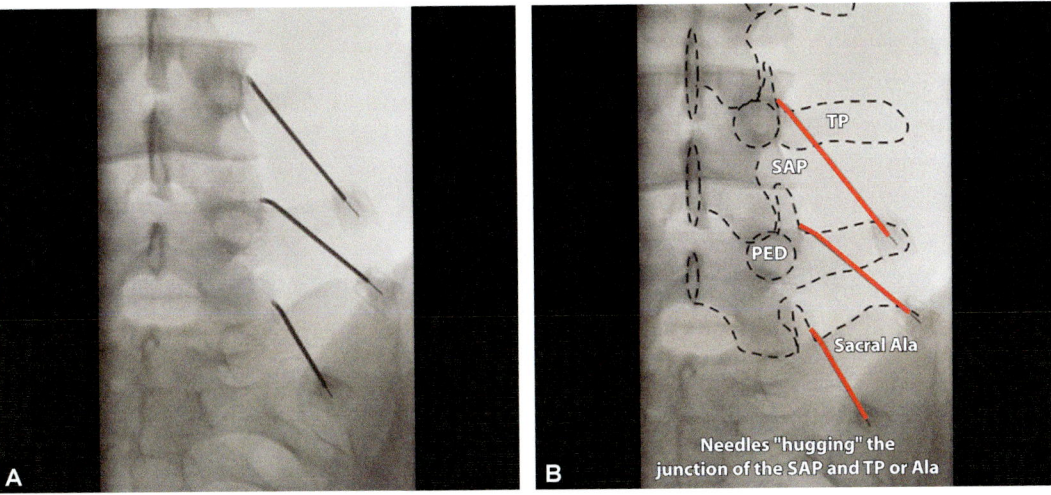

Figs. 6.21A and B: (A) Lumbar medial branch block—AP view. Final needle position; (B) Lumbar medial branch block—AP view. Final needle position (labeled).

PROVOCATIVE LUMBAR DISCOGRAPHY

Indication
Axial back pain presumably related to disc pathology

Advantages
- Diagnostic evaluation to determine the pain generating disc
- This technique can also be used to perform a thoracic discography as well.

Disadvantages/Complications
- Literature has shown that discs exposed to needle punctures may experience an accelerated disc degeneration, disc herniation, and loss of disc height compared to control groups[2]
- Discitis
- Increased pain

Techniques (Similar to an Infraneural TFESI)
1. *Pre-procedure:* Administer weight-based antibiotic prophylaxis (i.e. IV Cefazolin 2–3 g)
2. *Patient position:* Prone
3. *Target:* Middle 1/3 of the disc in AP and lateral views
   - At least 2 discs to be tested (control and suspected pathologic disc)
4. *AP view:* Square off vertebral body at level of injection, ensure spinous process is equidistant between pedicles
5. *Oblique view:* Rotate ipsilateral 35–45° or until SAP bisects disc
6. Advance spinal needle (5–8" × 22–25 g) toward a location 2–3 mm lateral to the upper 2/3rd of SAP
   - *Needle-in-needle technique:* Use a shorter, larger gauge needle as a guide; advance the larger needle close to the upper 2/3rd of the SAP and remove the stylet when approaching or passing by the facet. Then introduce the longer, smaller gauge needle, with a curved tip, through the outer needle and aim toward the center of the disc in both an AP and cranio-caudal dimension. This reduces chance of disc infection. You can pair an 3.5 inch, 18 g needle with a 5–8 inch 22 g needle; or use a 20 g/25 g combo.

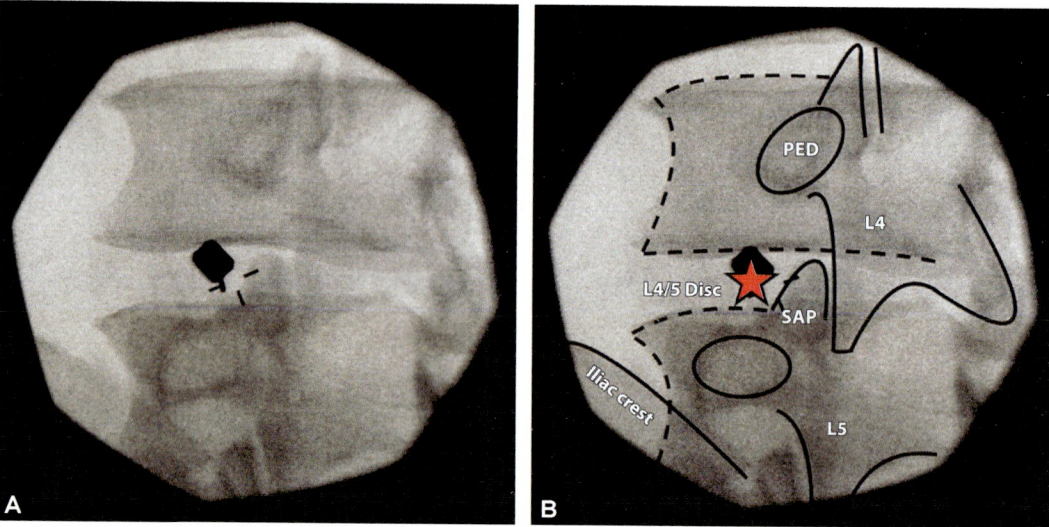

Figs. 6.22A and B: (A) Lumbar discography—35–45° ipsilateral rotation or until the superior articular process (SAP) bisects the vertebral body; (B) Lumbar discography—ipsilateral rotation (labeled).

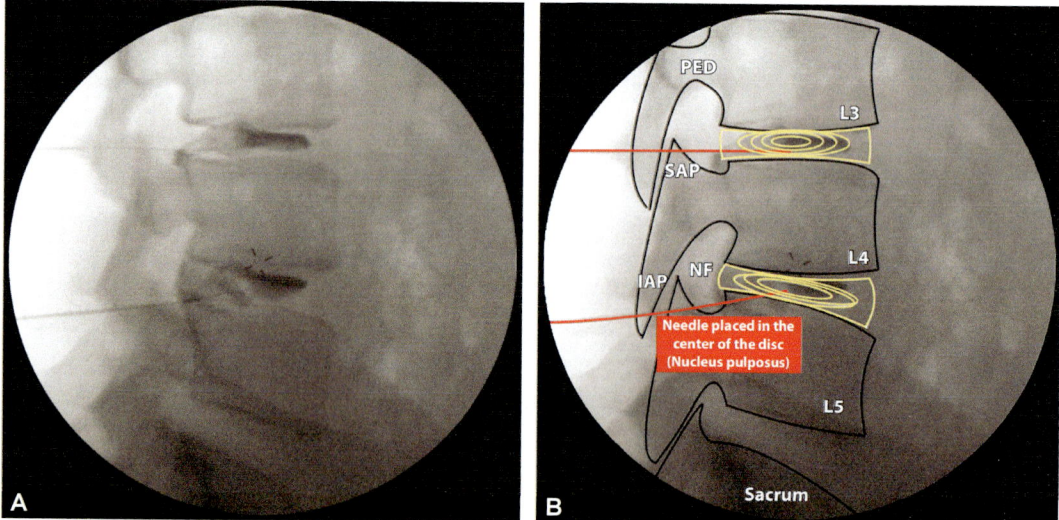

Figs. 6.23A and B: (A) Lumbar discography—lateral view. Needle advanced to the middle of the disc; (B) Lumbar discography—lateral view (labeled).

7. Periodically check AP and lateral views with every 1–1.5 cm advancement
   - Needle should rest in the middle of the disc corresponding to the spinous process
   - If the needle is not moving anterior at same rate as moving medially, needle is aimed too medially. Converse is true if needle not moving as medial as expected.
8. Obtain opening pressure: using an appropriate disc manometry device
   - Slowly begin to inject nonionic radiopaque contrast mixed with 1–10 mg/ml of Cefalozin until pain is elicited or until the pressure is greater than 100 psi (max 3 ml).

Chapter 6: Lumbar Spine, Hips and Lower Extremities

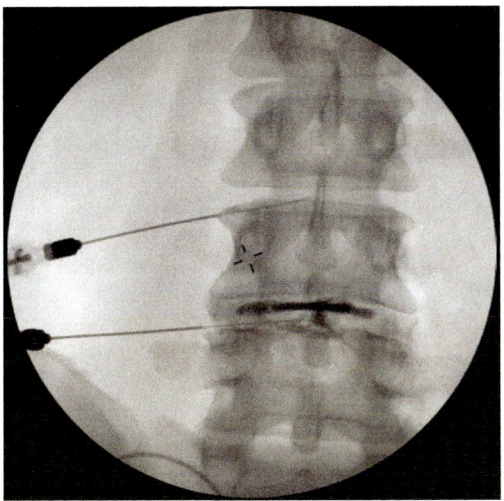

Fig. 6.24: Lumbar discography—AP view. Needle confirmed to be at the center of the disc. 1.5 cc of contrast producing a nucleogram.

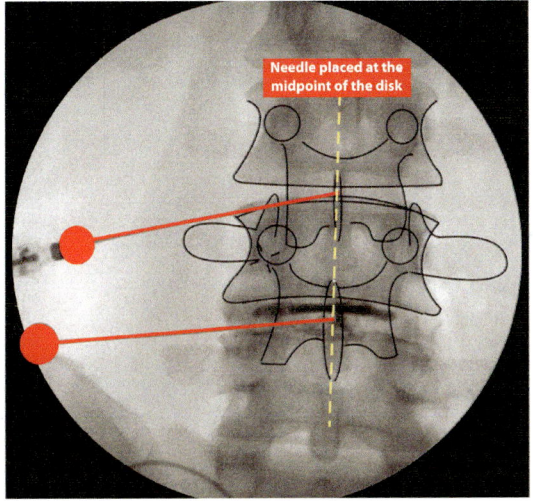

Fig. 6.25: Lumbar discography—AP view. Contrast with cotton ball appears. No gross signs of degeneration.

Target volume may be up to 2–3 cc maximum, though less can be injected if an answer is apparent.
9. *CT scan*: Post-procedure, to determine Dallas grade
   - Ensure cross sections are obtained by specifying that scan is for disc evaluation

SPINAL CORD STIMULATOR TRIAL—LUMBAR
Indications
- Patients who have failed interventions and conservative management.

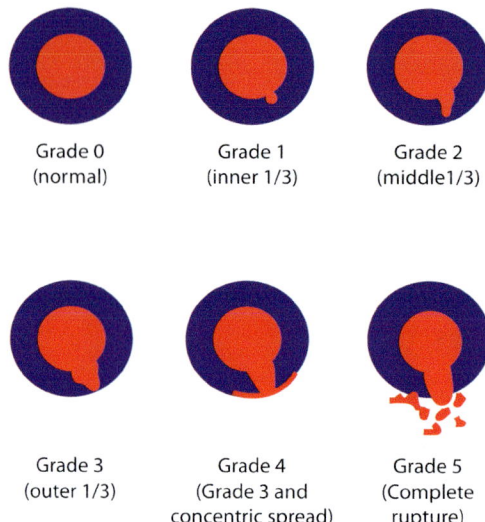

Fig. 6.26: Lumbar discography—Modified Dallas discogram classification. A system based approach that rates the degree of annular tearing, as seen on axial CT scans, following intradiskal contrast administration.[3]

- Lumbar radiculopathy ± axial back pain, complex regional pain syndrome, painful peripheral neuropathies.
- Failed back syndrome.

Advantages
- Direct stimulation of the dorsal column can cause changes within the ascending sensory fibers that modulate the intensity of painful stimuli.
- Potential for long-term benefits.
- Steroid sparing.

Disadvantages/Complications
- Lead migration, lead fracture, discomfort with paresthesia.
- *Standard ESI risks*: Unintended dural puncture with PDPH, infection, hematomas, nerve injury, spinal cord infarct, worsening pain, etc.
- Need for ongoing magnetic resonance imaging (MRI) is conditional based upon device.
- Contraindicated in patients with implanted cardiac defibrillators.

Techniques
1. *Preprocedure*: Administer prophylactic weight-based antibiotics (i.e. IV cefazolin 2–3 g).
2. *Patient position*: Prone with pillows under the abdomen to minimize lordosis.
3. *Target*: L1/L2 or L2/L3 epidural interspace.
4. *Anteroposterior view*: Square off the respective vertebral body and ensure spinous process is midline.
5. Start by placing the epidural introducer needle just lateral to the pedicle 1 level below the level of entrance (approx. 20–30° angle from midline). This directs the lead midline upon epidural access and the shallow angle facilitates lead steering (Figs. 6.27A and B).
   ◊ Advance toward midline of the targeted interspace
   ◊ The needle should be advanced at a 30–45° angle from the skin.

Chapter 6: Lumbar Spine, Hips and Lower Extremities

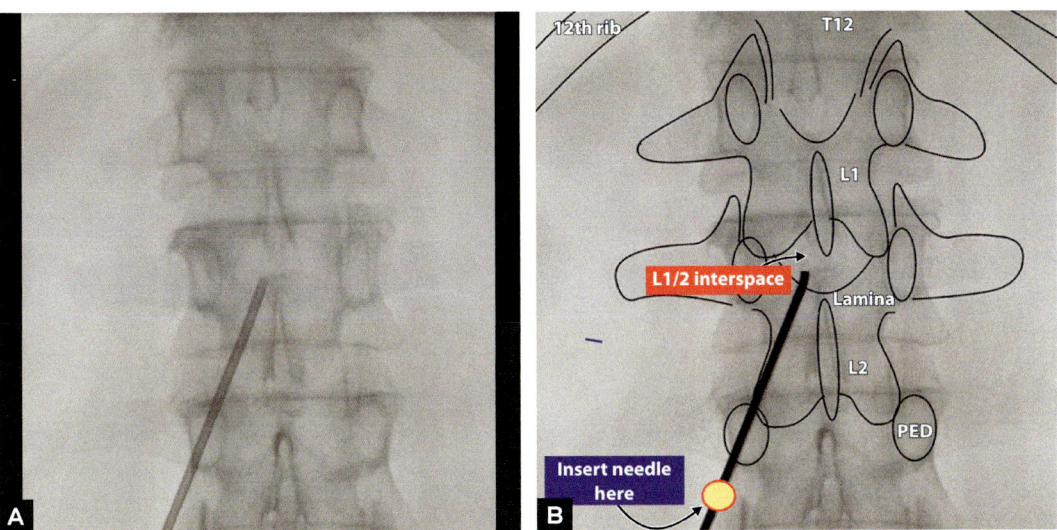

Figs. 6.27A and B: (A) Spinal cord stimulator (SCS) trial lumbar—AP view. Place the epidural introducer needle just lateral to the pedicle one level below the level of entrance (approx. 20–30° angle from midline); (B) SCS trial lumbar—AP view (labeled).

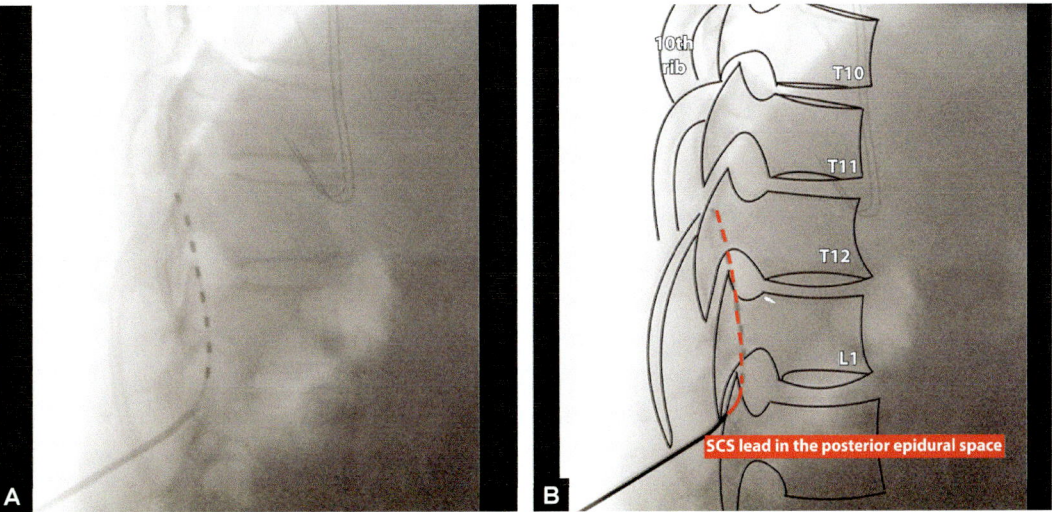

Figs. 6.28A and B: (A) Spinal cord stimulator trial lumbar—lateral view. Leads in the posterior epidural space; (B) Spinal cord stimulator trial lumbar—lateral view (labeled).

6. Contact the edge of the lower lamina and walk off superiorly
   ◊ Connect the LOR syringe to needle
   ◊ Advance toward midline until LOR occurs.
7. Thread lead through the introducer needle and advance lead in midline position to T8–T10 vertebral bodies.
8. *Lateral view*: Confirm placement in posterior epidural space (Figs. 6.28A and B). Difficult or painful advancement may reflect lateral/anterior placement or scar tissue.
9. Adjust leads based on stimulation test (Figs. 6.29A and B; Table 6.1).

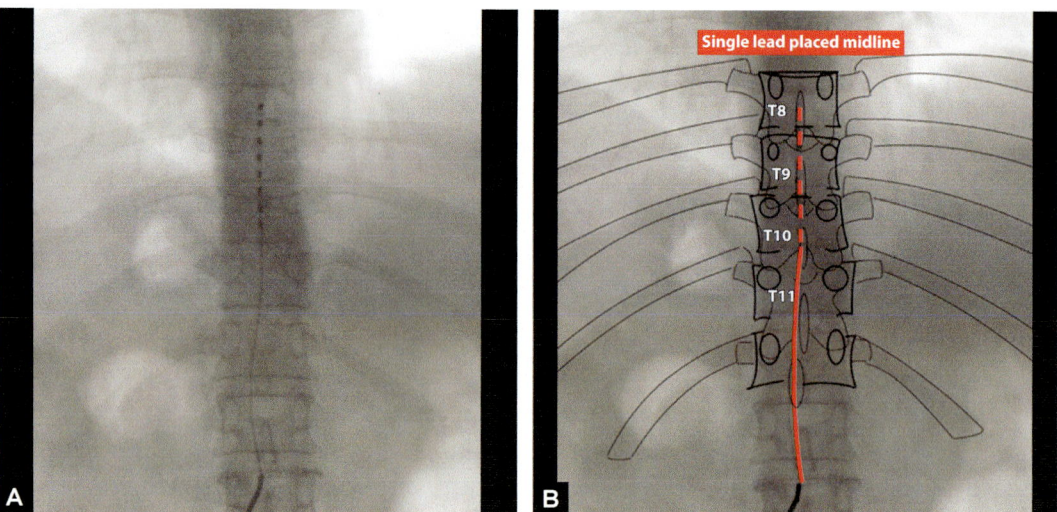

Figs. 6.29A and B: (A) Spinal cord stimulator trial lumbar—AP view with lead placement; (B) Spinal cord stimulator trial lumbar—AP view with lead placement (labeled).

Table 6.1: Lead placement along specific target areas.[4]	
Lead placement	Target areas
T5 to T6	Abdomen
T7 to T9	Back and legs
T11 to T12	Pelvis

10. A second parallel lead may be required if pain is bilateral and not covered by a single lead. If so, the leads should be placed 2–3 mm lateral on each side of midline.

INTRATHECAL TRIAL—LUMBAR

Indications
- Patients who have failed interventions and conservative management.
- Greater than 50% relief from systemic opioids but limited by side effects.
- Spasticity.
- Neuropathic and nociceptive pain.

Advantages
- Potential for long-term benefits.
- Intrathecal (IT) therapy allows targeted delivery to the spinal cord with much reduced central side effects (Table 6.2).

Disadvantages/Complications
- Postdural puncture headache, infection, hematomas, meningitis, orthostatic hypotension, respiratory depression, urinary retention.
- Prior opioids—wean before or not?
- Debatable—epidural versus IT, bolus versus continuous infusion
- Hospital admission during a continuous infusion trial.

Chapter 6: Lumbar Spine, Hips and Lower Extremities

Table 6.2: Recommended intrathecal (IT) bolus dose.[5]

Drug	Recommended intrathecal (IT) bolus dose
Morphine	0.2–1.0 mg
Hydromorphone	0.04–0.2 mg
Ziconotide	1–5 µg
Fentanyl	25–75 µg
Bupivacaine	0.5–2.5 mg
Clonidine	5–20 µg
Sufentanil	5–20 µg
Baclofen	50–100 µg

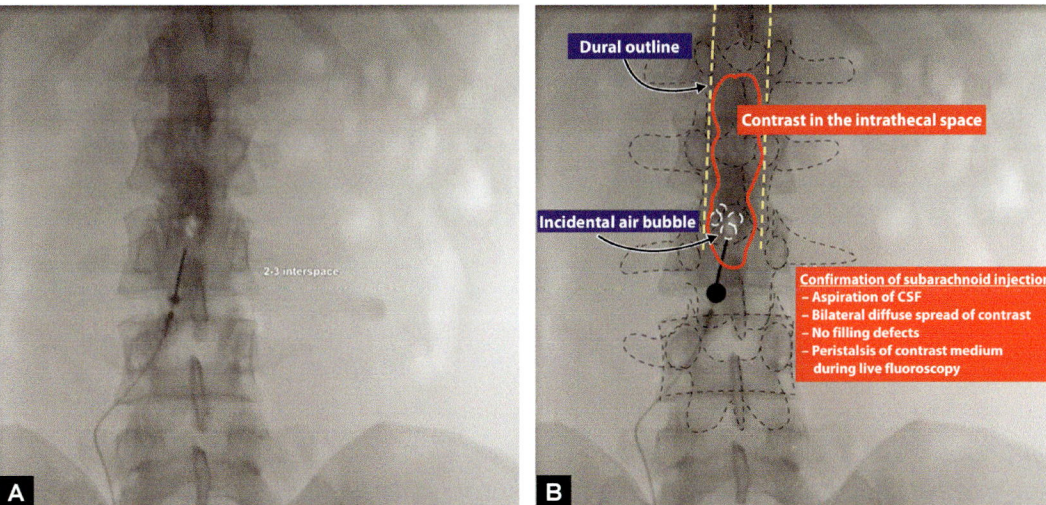

Figs. 6.30A and B: (A) Intrathecal trial—AP view with contrast in the intrathecal space; (B) Intrathecal trial—AP view with contrast in the intrathecal space (labeled).

Techniques

1. *Patient position*: Prone with pillows under the abdomen to minimize lordosis.
2. *Target*: L1/L2 interspace or below.
3. *Anteroposterior view*: Square off the respective vertebral body and ensure spinous process is midline (Figs. 6.30A and B).
    ◊ Using a 3.5 inch × 22 G spinal needle, advance toward midline of the interspace.
    ◊ As the ligamentum flavum and dura are transversed, a change in resistance is noted, "a pop". Once in the subarachnoid space, remove the stylet and cerebrospinal fluid (CSF) should appear.
4. *Lateral view*: Confirm placement in the IT space (Figs. 6.31A and B).
5. Proceed to implant, after passing a psychological screen, if:
    ◊ *Baclofen*: Reduction in spasticity greater than 30% (Modified Ashworth scale decreased by 1) and/or demonstrates improvement in function or pain.
    ◊ *Opioids*: Greater than 50% relief.

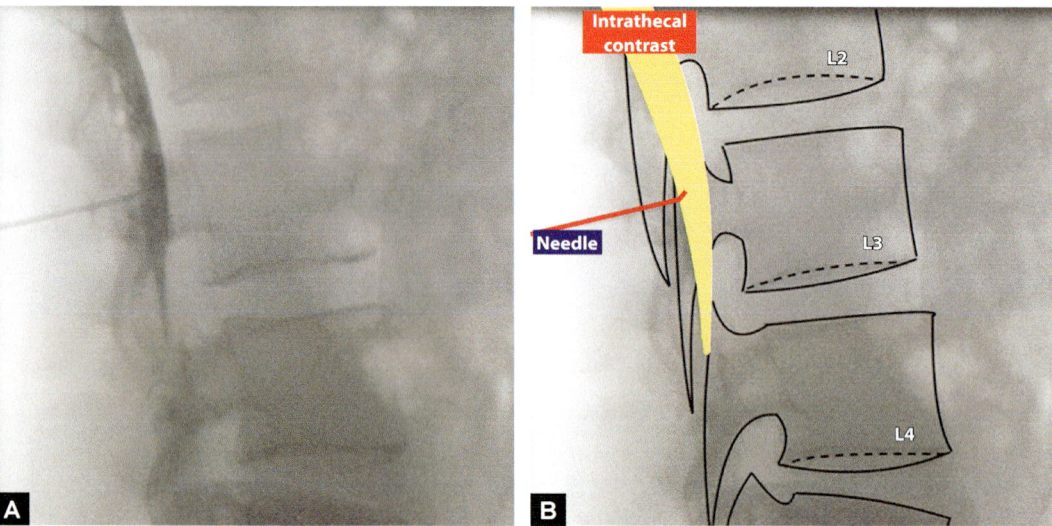

Figs. 6.31A and B: (A) Intrathecal trial—lateral view with contrast; (B) Intrathecal trial—lateral view. Contrast producing a convex appearance (thick in the center compared to the edges)—labeled.

SACROILIAC JOINT INJECTION: INFERIOR APPROACH

Indication
Diagnostic and/or therapeutic treatment for sacroiliac joint (SIJ) pain.

Advantages
- Minimal risk.
- Can easily supplement intra-articular injection with periarticular injection as surrounding ligaments can also be pain generators.

Disadvantages/Complications
- Innervation to the SIJ is debatable (primarily S1, S2; L5, S3, S4 and the ventral contributions is variable).
- Multiple approaches to the joint and none are superior to the others.
- Anterior leakage of injectate into pelvis can cause a lumbosacral block.

Injectate
1 mL steroid of choice + 1 mL bupivacaine 0.5%.

Techniques
1. *Patient position*: Prone.
2. *Target*: Inferior aspect of the posterior SIJ.
3. *Anteroposterior view*: Identify the anterior and posterior joint lines.
    ◊ The posterior SIJ appears medial (S-shaped) to the anterior portion.
4. *Optimize view (Figs. 6.32A and B)*: Tilt cephalad 10–15° and rotate ipsilateral less than 10°.
    ◊ This improves the lucency of the inferior portion of the posterior joint.

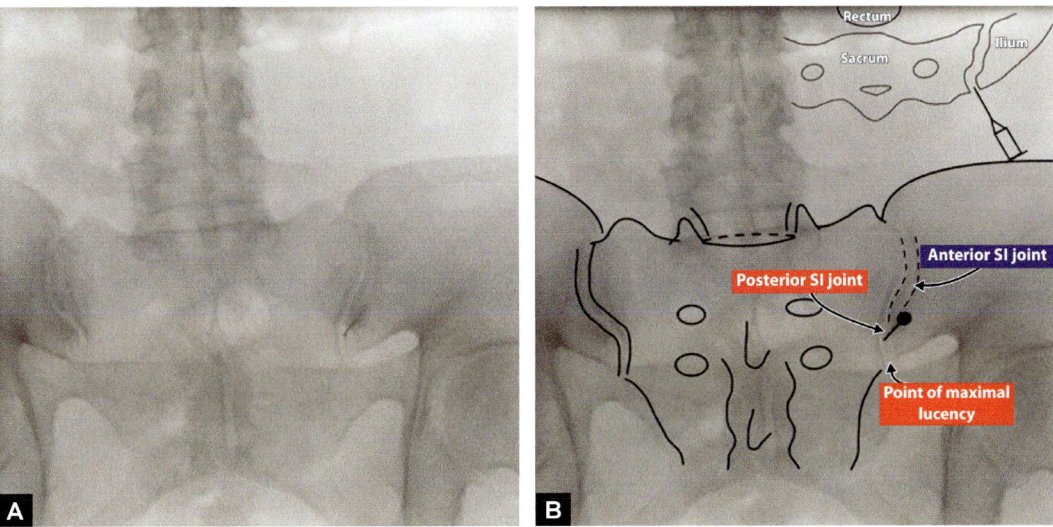

Figs. 6.32A and B: (A) Sacroiliac joint (SIJ) injection: identify the inferior portion of the joint. Tilt cephalad 10–15° and rotate ipsilateral 5–10° to optimize the lucency of the inferior portion of the joint; (B) SIJ injection: oblique angulation. The posterior SIJ will be medial to the anterior SIJ (labeled).

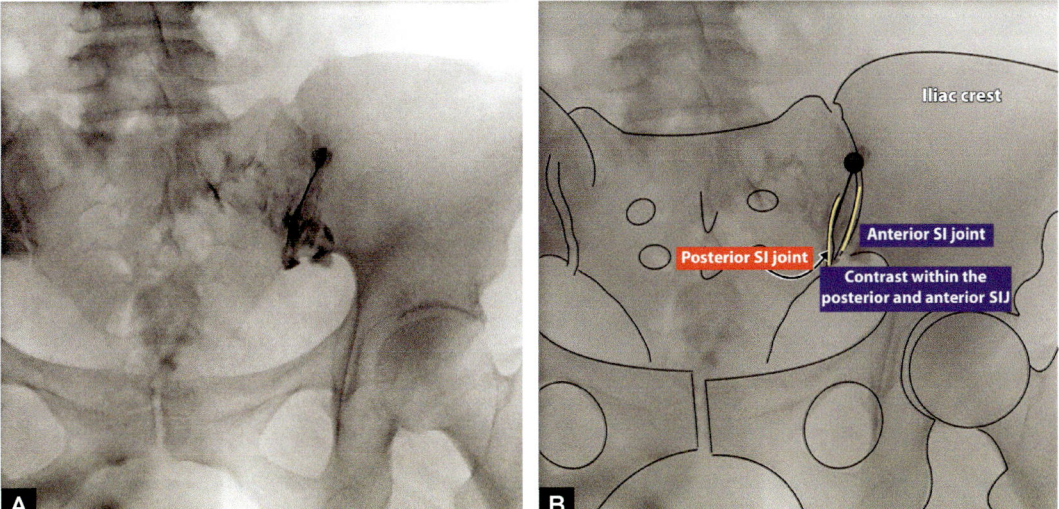

Figs. 6.33A and B: (A) Sacroiliac joint injection: contrast spread; (B) SIJ injection: contrast spread. The SIJ can hold less than 2 mL of volume (labeled).

5. Advance spinal needle (3.5–6 inch × 22–25 G) toward the inferior aspect.
   ◊ Target the lucent portion (normally 0.5–1 cm above the most inferior portion) until the needle contacts the sacrum or enters into the joint capsule (eraser-like consistency).
   ◊ Walk off the sacrum from medial to lateral until the needle enters the joint.
6. Confirm in contralateral/lateral views (Figs. 6.33 and 6.34).

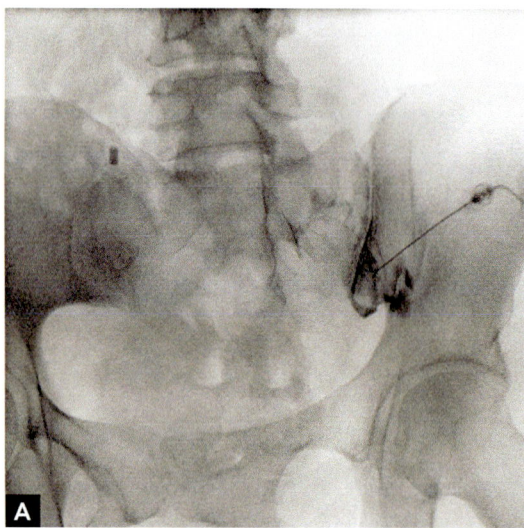 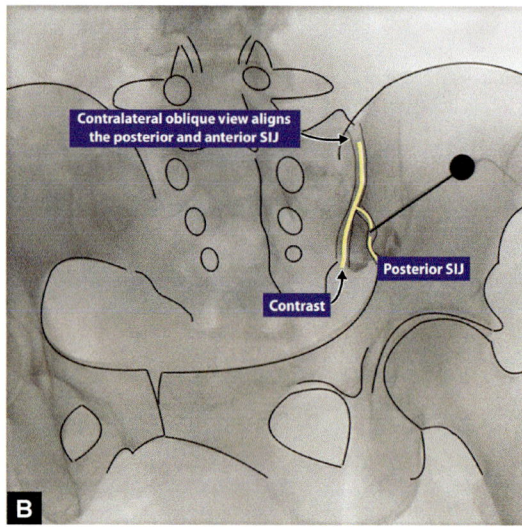

Figs. 6.34A and B: (A) Sacroiliac joint injection: contralateral oblique view (5–15°). The contralateral oblique view aligns the posterior and anterior joint lines. Utilizing this view can enhance your visualized of contrast spread; (B) Sacroiliac joint injection: contralateral oblique view (5–15°). Contrast spread (labeled).

DORSAL RAMI (L5) AND LATERAL BRANCH BLOCKS (S1-S3)

Indication
Diagnostic and/or therapeutic treatment for SIJ pain.

Advantages
- Utilized when a successful diagnostic/therapeutic SIJ injection provides only short-term relief.
- Option to proceed to RFA (traditional vs cooled) to provide long-lasting relief.

Disadvantage/Complication
Innervation to the SIJ is debatable (primarily S1, S2, L5, S3, S4 and the ventral contributions is variable).

Injectate
0.5–1 mL bupivacaine 0.5% per site.

Techniques
1. *Patient position*: Prone
2. *Targets*:
    ◊ *L5 DR*: Junction of the L5 SAP and the sacral ala.
    ◊ *S1-S3 lateral branches*: 1 cm lateral to the respective foramen.
3. *Anteroposterior view*: Identify the junction of the SAP and the sacral ala.
4. *Optimize view*: Tilt caudal 5° and oblique ipsilateral 5° (Fig. 6.35).
5. Advance spinal needle (3.5-6 inch × 22-25 G) toward the SAP and ala junction. Contact the ala and walk off 1-2 mm.

Chapter 6: Lumbar Spine, Hips and Lower Extremities

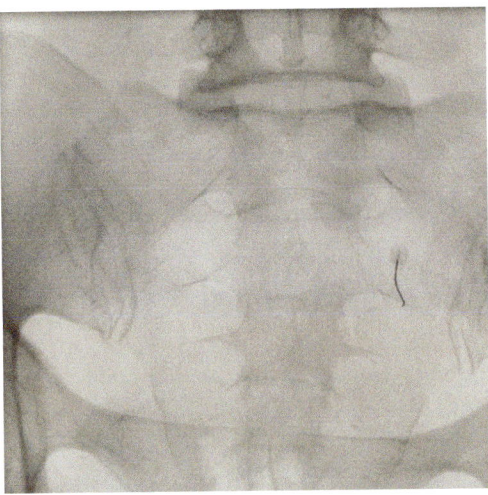

Fig. 6.35: Lateral branch block (S1-S3)—AP view. To help identify the foramen, tilt caudal and oblique ipsilateral 5°.

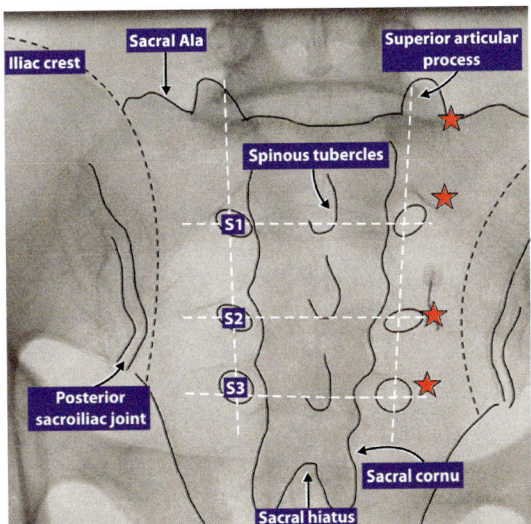

Fig. 6.36: Lateral branch block (S1-S3)—AP view. To assist with the identification of the foramens, draw a vertical line at the midpoint of the L5 pedicle or the facet joint. Then draw a horizontal line across the spinous tubercles. They intersect at each foramen (labeled).

6. *Anteroposterior view*: Identify the S1-S3 foramens (Fig. 6.36).
   ◊ Foramens align with the facet joint lines superiorly and the sacral spinous tubercles laterally
   ◊ Locations will be symmetric to contralateral foramen.
7. Target approximately 1 cm lateral to the foramens until the sacrum is contacted.
8. Lateral view to confirm depth and that needle is not in or past the foramen.
9. Confirm placement with contrast.

LUMBAR SYMPATHETIC BLOCK

Indication
Sympathetically mediated pain conditions such as lower extremity chronic regional pain syndrome (CRPS), ischemic pain such as from peripheral vascular disease, phantom limb pain, or neuropathic pain.

Advantages
- Provides diagnostic and therapeutic value.
- For prolonged benefits, chemoneurolysis or RFA can be performed.

Disadvantages/Complications
- Risk of epidural or intrathecal injection, toxic levels of local anesthetics given high volume, hematuria or direct needle placement in the kidney which is self-limited (higher risk at L2 level).
- When performed bilaterally, higher chance of hypotension, priapism and diarrhea.

Injectate
40–80 mg of methylprednisolone or steroid of choice + 15 mL bupivacaine 0.25–0.5%.

Techniques
1. *Patient position*: Prone
2. *Target*: Inferior portion of the anterior one-third of the L2, L3, or L4 vertebral body.
3. *Anteroposterior view*: Square off vertebral body (L2, L3, or L4) at level of injection.
4. *Oblique view*: Rotate ipsilateral until the tip of the TP is aligned the vertebral body (usually 25–35°) (Figs. 6.37A and B).
5. Advance spinal needle (5–6 inch × 22 G) toward target level. The ganglia lie between L2-L4.
    ◊ Maintain needle tip in contact with the vertebral body so as not to stray too lateral.
6. *Lateral view*: Confirm depth and that the final position is at the anterior one-third of the vertebral body.
7. Confirm placement with contrast in both AP and lateral views (Figs. 6.38 and 6.39).
    ◊ If the psoas muscle is outline, the needle may be too lateral and the needle must be pulled back and redirected medially. It may also be too superficial and need to be advanced further but not beyond the anterior border of the vertebral body.
8. Successful block should yield an increase in temperature by at least 2°C and decrease in pain if sympathetically maintained. Temperature cannot increase above core body. If there is a successful temperature change however no pain relief, patient may be sympathetically independent pain.

INTRA-ARTICULAR HIP INJECTION

Indication
Hip pain, hip osteoarthritis.

Advantages
- Safe and accurate placement of steroids compared to blind or ultrasound-guided techniques.
- A greater and lesser trochanter bursa injection can also be easily supplemented.

Chapter 6: Lumbar Spine, Hips and Lower Extremities

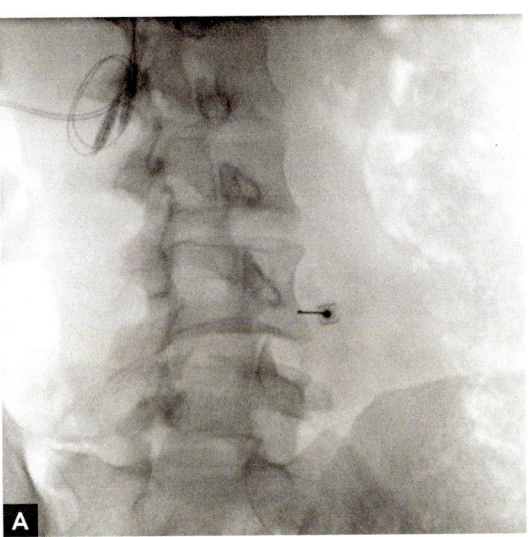 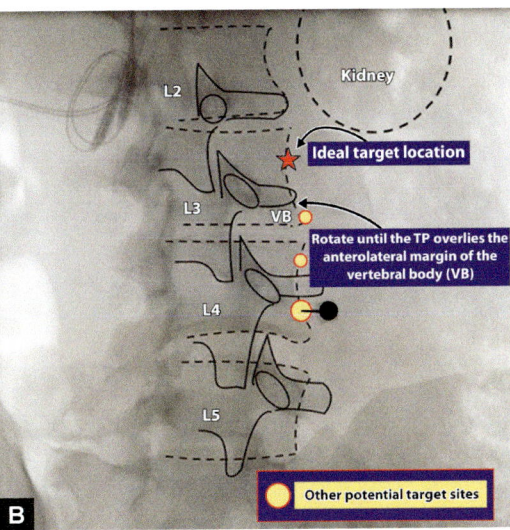

Figs. 6.37A and B: (A) Lumbar sympathetic block—ipsilateral rotation 25–30° or until the transverse process is at anterolateral margin of the vertebral body. The sympathetic ganglia span L2-L4 where the largest portion around the L2/L3 disk. In order to avoid the kidney, perform the block at either L3 or L4. Performing the block below the transverse process carries the risk of nerve root penetration; (B) Lumbar sympathetic block—ipsilateral rotation 25–30° (labeled).

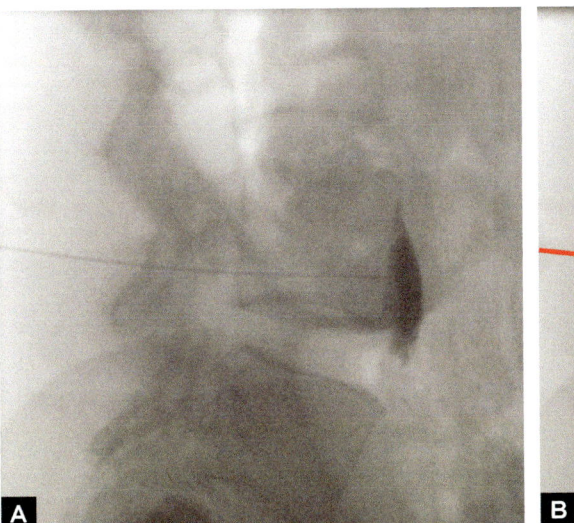 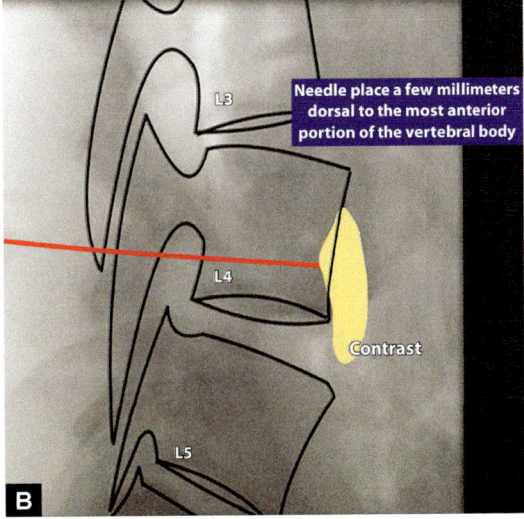

Figs. 6.38A and B: (A) Lumbar sympathetic block—lateral view with contrast. Needle tip placed at the anterior one-third or a few millimeters dorsal to the most anterior portion of the vertebral body; (B) Lumbar sympathetic block—lateral view with contrast (labeled).

Disadvantages/Complications
- Neurovascular injection.
- Periarticular injection causing a femoral nerve block.

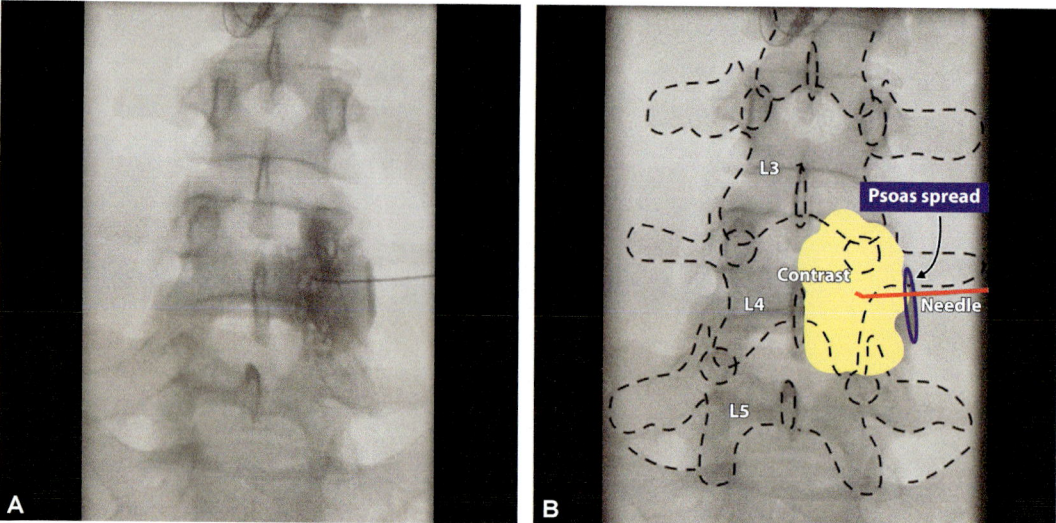

Figs. 6.39A and B: (A) Lumbar sympathetic block—AP view with contrast; (B) Lumbar sympathetic block—AP view with contrast (labeled).

- Multiple steroid injections can have deleterious effect on cartilage, cause bone loss, osteoporosis, osteonecrosis.

Injectate
40 mg of methylprednisolone or steroid of choice + 3–4 mL of bupivacaine 0.25–0.5%.

Techniques
1. *Patient position*: Supine
2. *Target*: Intracapsular location on the mid-femoral neck.
3. *Anteroposterior view*: Identify the femoral neck.
4. Advance spinal needle (3.5 inch × 22–25 G) toward the target.
5. Once osseous contact is made, withdraw slightly and advance the needle further superiorly to gain entrance to the capsule.
6. Confirm placement with contrast in AP view. The arthrogram should display a circumferential spread (Figs. 6.40A and B).

ARTICULAR BRANCH BLOCKS OF THE FEMORAL AND OBTURATOR NERVES
Indication
Hip pain, hip osteoarthritis, pain s/p hip arthroplasty.

Advantages
- Provides diagnostic information and if successful can proceed to RFA or chemoneurolysis for longer relief. These are pure sensory branches of the femoral and obturator nerves.
- Steroid sparing.

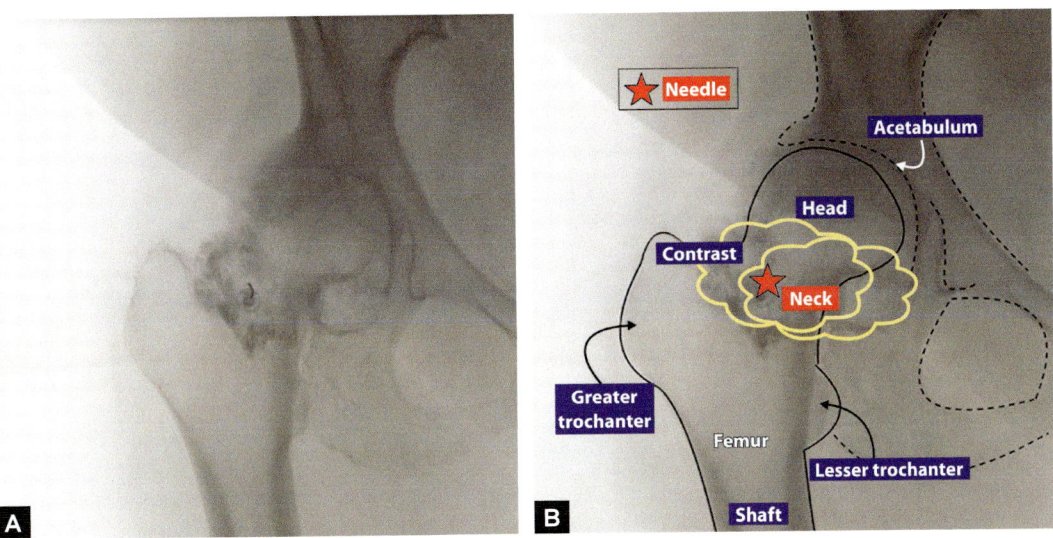

Figs. 6.40A and B: (A) Intra-articular hip injection—AP view with contrast; (B) Intra-articular hip injection—AP view with contrast (labeled).

Disadvantage/Complication
Neurovascular injection, leg weakness, numbness in the groin or leg.

Injectate
2–3 mL of bupivacaine 0.5% ± 20 mg of methylprednisolone or steroid of choice.

Techniques
1. *Patient position*: Prone.
2. *Target*:
   ◊ *Femoral articular branch*: Just medial to the anterior inferior iliac spine (AIIS).
   ◊ *Obturator articular branch*: Incisura of the acetabulum.
3. *Anteroposterior view*: Tilt caudal 10–15°, rotate ipsilateral 5° (Figs. 6.41A and B).
4. Advance spinal needle (3.5 inch × 22–25 G) toward the respective targets until osseous contact is made.
5. Confirm placement with contrast.
6. Repeat process for other articular branch.

INTRA-ARTICULAR KNEE INJECTION
Indication
Knee pain, knee osteoarthritis.

Advantage
Safe and accurate placement of steroids compared to blind or ultrasound-guided techniques.

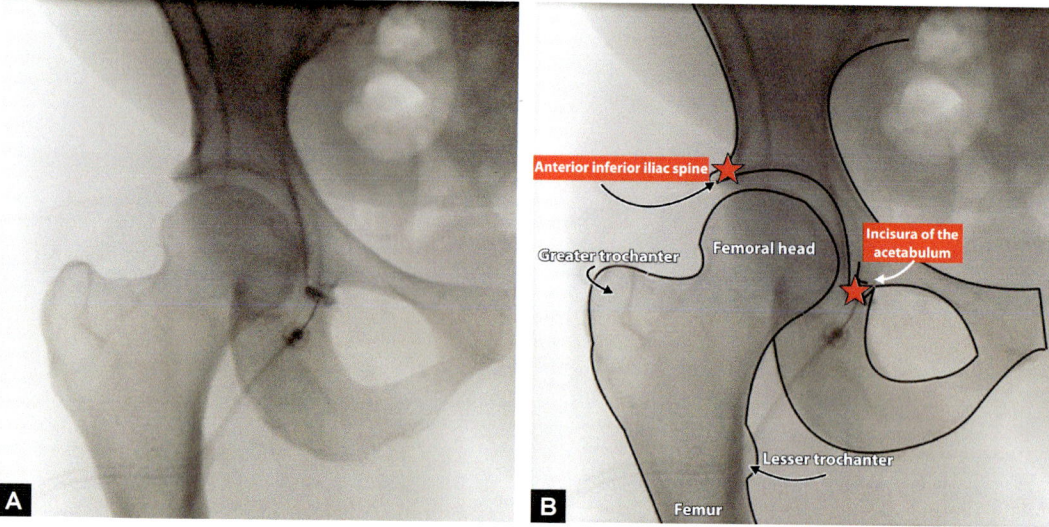

Figs. 6.41A and B: (A) Articular branch blocks of the femoral and obturator nerves—tilt caudal 10–15°, rotate ipsilateral 5°. Target the anterior inferior iliac spine (for femoral branch) and the incisura of the acetabulum (Contrast shown here is at the incisura for an obturator branch block.); (B) Articular branch blocks of the femoral and obturator nerves. Target the anterior inferior iliac spine and the incisura of the acetabulum (labeled).

Disadvantages/Complications
- Neurovascular injection.
- Multiple steroid injections can have deleterious effect on cartilage, cause bone loss, osteoporosis, osteonecrosis.

Injectate
40 mg of methylprednisolone + 3–4 mL of bupivacaine 0.25–0.5%.

Techniques
1. *Patient position*: Supine with knee in slight flexion.
2. *Target*: Lateral compartment of the knee joint.
3. *Anteroposterior view*: Identify the lateral compartment of the knee (Figs. 6.42A and B).
4. Advance needle (1.5–3.5 inch × 22–25G) lateral to medial toward the target until the needle lies in the middle of the compartment.
5. Confirm placement with contrast. The arthrogram should spread to the contralateral compartment.

KNEE GENICULAR NERVE BLOCKS (FOUR LOCATIONS)
Indications
- Knee pain (theoretically better results for anterior pain).
- Knee osteoarthritis.
- S/p total knee arthroplasty.

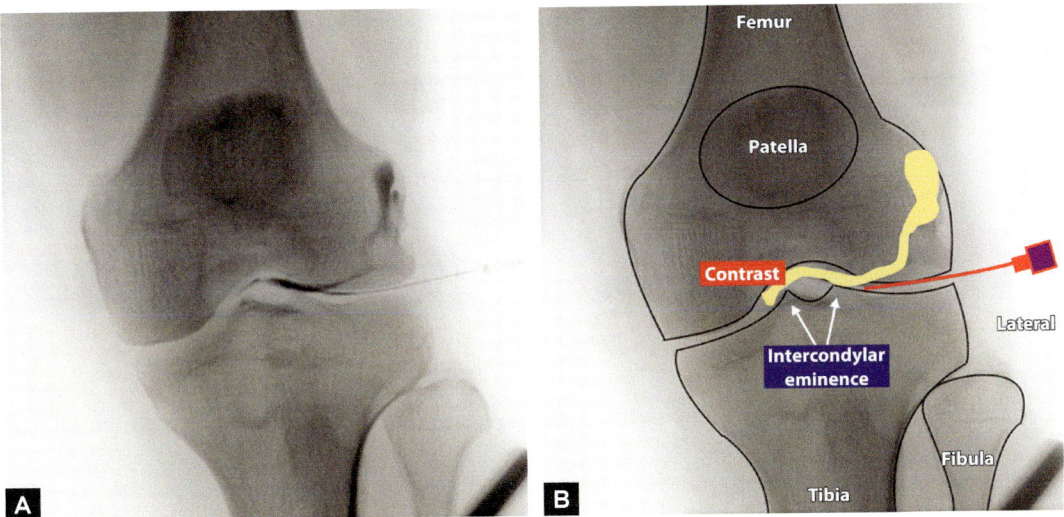

Figs. 6.42A and B: (A) Knee intra-articular injection—AP view; (B) Knee intra-articular injection—AP view (labeled).

Advantages
- Genicular nerves are sensory branches of the obturator, tibial, common fibular and femoral nerves. Therefore, this procedure provides diagnostic information and therapeutic benefit.
- If successful, can proceed to RFA.
- Steroid sparing.

Disadvantage/Complication
Complete block to the knee joint cannot be achieved without motor block due to proximity of sensory branches to parent nerve. The nerves to be avoided include (1) inferolateral branch of the fibular nerve due to risk of foot drop and the (2) posterior sensory nerves.

Injectate
1–2 mL of bupivacaine 0.25–0.5% ± 40 mg methylprednisolone or steroid of choice divided between the injection sites.

Techniques
1. *Patient position*: Supine with knee in extension.
2. *Targets*: Genicular branches typically located *near inflection points* (between shaft and condyle) at a depth of approximately one-half to two-thirds of the shaft width.
    ◊ *Distal femur*: Medial
    ◊ *Distal femur*: Lateral
    ◊ *Proximal tibia*: Medial
    ◊ *Suprapatella (optional)*: Approximately 3–4 cm above the patella (femoral nerve supplies branches to the three vasti and small branches to innervate part of the joint).
3. *Anteroposterior view*: Identify the four regions (Figs. 6.43A and B).

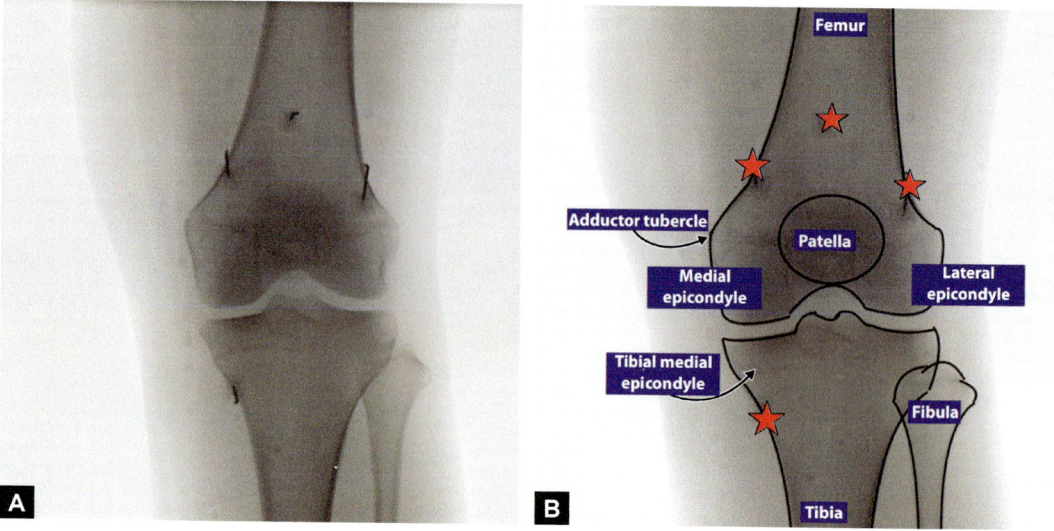

Figs. 6.43A and B: (A) Genicular nerve block—AP view; (B) Genicular nerve block—AP view (labeled).

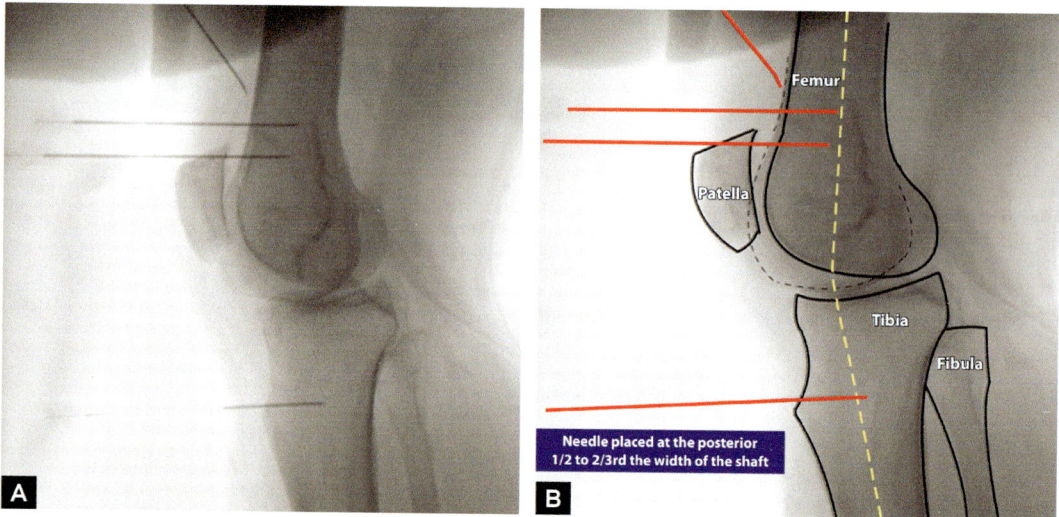

Figs. 6.44A and B: (A) Genicular nerve block—lateral view; (B) Genicular nerve block—lateral view (labeled).

4. Advance spinal needle (3.5 inch × 22–25 G) toward the target location until osseous contact is made.
5. *Lateral view*: Advance needle until it lies at one-half to two-thirds depth of the shaft (Figs. 6.44A and B).
6. Confirm placement with contrast. Repeat process for remaining nerves.

REFERENCES

1. Bogduk N. Practice Guidelines for Spinal Diagnostic and Treatment Procedures, 2nd edition. San Francisco: International Spine Intervention Society; 2013.

2. Carragee EJ, Don AS, Hurwitz EL, et al. 2009 ISSLS Prize Winner: Does discography cause accelerated progression of degeneration changes in the lumbar disc: a ten-year matched cohort study. Spine (Phila Pa 1976). 2009;34:2338-45.
3. Sachs BL, Vanharanta H, Spivey MA, et al. Dallas discogram description. A new classification of CT/discography in low-back disorders. Spine (Phila Pa 1976). 1987;12:287-94
4. Deer TR. Atlas of Implantable Therapies for Pain Management. New York: Springer Science+Business Media; 2010.
5. Deer TR, Prager J, Levy R, et al. Polyanalgesic Consensus Conference—2012: recommendations on trialing for intrathecal (intraspinal) drug delivery: report of an interdisciplinary expert panel. Neuromodulation. 2012;15(5):420-35; discussion 435.

HALL OF REFERENCES

In some form or fashion, I have adopted or modified a technique from one of these sources. These books were highly utilized during my training, so I must acknowledge and say thank you all for your contribution to my education.
1. Bogduk N. Practice Guidelines for Spinal Diagnostic and Treatment Procedures, 2nd edition, San Francisco: International Spine Intervention Society; 2014.
2. Furman MB, Lee TS, Berkwits L. Atlas of Image-Guided Spinal Procedures. Philadelphia: Elsevier Saunders; 2013.
3. Rathmell JP. Atlas of Image-Guided Intervention in Regional Anesthesia and Pain Medicine. Philadelphia: Lippincott Williams & Wilkins; 2006.
4. Waldman SD. Atlas of Interventional Pain Management, 3rd edition. Philadelphia: Elsevier Saunders; 2009.
5. Waldman SD. Atlas of Interventional Pain Management, 4th edition. Philadelphia: Elsevier Saunders; 2015.
6. Narouze SN. Interventional Management of Head and Face Pain. New York: Springer; 2014.

Index

Page numbers followed by f refer to figure.

A

Abdomen 38
Accidental cerebrospinal fluid 17*f*
Acetabulum, incisura of 86*f*
Anterior inferior iliac spine 7, 85
Antibiotics, administer 32
Aorta 48*f*
    anterolateral wall of 48*f*
Aortic penetration 45
Apixaban 9
Articular pillars 27*f*
    target midpoint of 22*f*
    target waist of 26*f*
Ashworth scale, modified 77
Aspiration 5
Aspirin 9
Atlantoaxial intra-articular injection 6, 24, 24*f*, 25*f*
Axial back pain 22, 25, 32, 40, 66, 68, 74

B

Baclofen 77
Betamethasone 12
Bilateral recurrent laryngeal nerves 35
Bisects vertebral body 72*f*
Bowel perforation 52
Brachial plexopathy 32
Bupivacaine 10, 15, 35, 77, 80, 85-87
Bursa 5

C

Carbocaine 10
Cardiac surgery 44
Cardiovascular toxicity 11
C-arm 1, 2*f*
Caudal epidural steroid injection 64
Cefazolin 32
Celiac plexus 4, 7
    block 45, 47, 47*f*, 48*f*

Central nervous system toxicity 10
Cephalad 1
Cephalic tilt 1
Cerebrospinal fluid aspiration 15
Cervical
    epidural steroid injection 28
    facet intra-articular injection 22, 22*f*, 23*f*
    interlaminar epidural steroid injection 28*f*, 29*f*
    lead placement 33
    medial branch block 25, 26*f*, 27*f*
    radiculopathy 28, 30, 32
    spinal
        cord stimulator trial 32*f*, 33*f*
        stenosis 28, 30
    spondylosis 22, 24, 25
    sympathetic 4
    transforaminal epidural
        steroid injection 6, 30, 30*f*
Chassaignac's tubercle 35
Chemoneurolysis 15, 27, 69
Chemoneurolytic ablation 25, 68
Chest wall pain 44
Christmas tree appearance 67*f*
Chronic regional pain syndrome 19, 82
Clonidine 77
Clopidogrel 9
Coccygeal nerve block 4, 7
Complex regional pain syndrome 32, 74
Contralateral oblique rotation 2
Craniofacial blocks 4

D

Dabigatran 9
Dallas discogram classification, modified 74*f*
Decadron 12
Depomedrol 12
Dexamethasone 15
    acetate 12
Dextrose 25

Diarrhea 45
Discography 5
Dorsal rami 80

E

Eagle's syndrome 21
Endometriosis 50
Enoxaparin 9
Epidural
    block 45
    blood patch 4
    spread 52
    steroid injection 7, 38
External auditory meatus 21*f*

F

Facet
    arthrosis 25, 40, 68
    column 27*f*
    injection 58
    joint 24f, 38*f*, 67, 68*f*-70*f*, 81*f*
        intra-articular 5
        radiofrequency ablation 5
Facial pain, treatment of 15
Failed back syndrome 74
Failed neck syndrome 32
Femoral nerve 7
    articular branch blocks of 84, 86*f*
    block 83
Fentanyl 77
Final needle position 71*f*
Fluoroscopic imaging chain, components of 1*f*
Fluoroscopy 1, 4, 5
Foramen
    ovale 16, 16*f*, 17
    posterior one-third of 59*f*

G

Gadolinium 13
Ganglion impar block 4, 52, 53*f*-55*f*
Gasserian ganglion block 15, 15*f*-17*f*
Genicular nerve 87
    block 7, 88*f*
Genitourinary pain 50
Glenohumeral
    intra-articular injection 36*f*
    joint injection 6
    shoulder intra-articular injection 35*f*
Glossopharyngeal
    nerve block 6, 20, 21*f*
    neuralgia 20
Glucocorticoids, selection of 11

H

Head 15
Headaches 19
    cervicogenic 22, 24, 25
    occipital 22, 24, 25
Hematomas 32, 43, 56, 58, 60, 62, 63
Heparin 9
Hip 56
    arthroplasty 84
    articular branches of 7
    intra-articular injection 7
    osteoarthritis 82, 84
    pain 82, 84
Horner's syndrome 35
Humeral head, target superolateral portion of 36*f*
Hydromorphone 77
Hypotension 11, 45, 50

I

Iliac artery 50
Infection 35
Intercoccygeal joint approach 52
Intercostal nerve 4
    block 6, 44, 44*f*
Interlaminar epidural steroid injections 4
Interventional pain procedures 9
Intradiscal injection 50
Intrathecal
    block 45
    bolus dose 77
    injection 50
    trial 7, 76
Intravascular injection 15, 44, 63
Ipsilateral rotation 45*f*, 47*f*, 61*f*, 62*f*, 64*f*, 65*f*, 68*f*, 72*f*

J

Joint 5
    inferior portion of 79*f*
    sacrococcygeal 52, 53*f*
    target lateral one-third of 24*f*

K

Kambin's triangle 63
Knee
    genicular nerve blocks 86
    intra-articular injection 7, 87*f*
    osteoarthritis 85, 86
    pain 85, 86
Kuntz's fibers 35

L

Lateral branch block 80, 81*f*
Lead placement 33*f*
Leg weakness 85
Lidocaine 10
Local anesthetic 10
    complications 10
    pharmacology 10
Longus colli muscle 34*f*
Lordosis 2
    of spine, degree of 56*f*
Lumbar
    discography 7, 72*f*, 74*f*
    facet
        intra-articular injection 68*f*, 69*f*
        joint injection 7
    interlaminar epidural steroid injection 56, 56*f*
    intra-articular facet joint injection 66
    medial branch block 7, 68, 70*f*, 71*f*
    radiculopathy 56, 58, 60, 62, 63
    spinal stenosis 56, 60, 62, 63
    spine 56
    spondylosis 66, 68
    stenosis, severe 64
    sympathetic block 4, 7, 82, 83*f*, 84*f*
    transforaminal epidural steroid
        injection 58, 59f, 60, 62, 63

M

Magnetic resonance imaging 74
Mastoid air cells 16*f*
Maxillary
    and mandibular nerve block 6, 18, 18*f*
    sinus 18*f*
        posterior wall of 16*f*
    teeth 19
Medial branch block 5, 25, 26*f*, 27, 40, 68, 69
Mepivacaine 10
Methylene blue 25
Methylprednisolone 12, 35, 57, 85, 86, 87
Mid axial back pain 38
Morphine 77
Multiple steroid injections 35, 86

N

Nasal mucosa, superior-lateral margin of 20*f*
Nausea 15
Neck pain 28, 30
Needle placement, location of 26*f*
Needle-in-needle technique 71
Nerve injury 32, 43, 56, 58, 60, 62, 63
Neurovascular injection 35, 83, *85*, 86
North American Spine Society 11

O

Obturator nerves 7
    articular branch blocks of 84, 86*f*
Opioids 77
Osteonecrosis 35, 86
Osteoporosis 35, 86

P

Pain 20
    abdominal 44
    colorectal 50
    exacerbation of 67
    neuropathic 34
Painful peripheral neuropathies 32, 74
Paresthesia 63
Pelvic
    pain, chronic 50
    viscera 52
Pelvis 50
Periarticular injection 83
Perineum 50
Peripheral nerve 4
    blocks 4
Petrous bone 17*f*
Phantom limb pain 34
Phenol 25
Phrenic nerves 35
Pneumothorax 44, 45, 45*f*
Post-dural puncture headache 19, 43, 56
Posterior joint margin 25*f*
Post-herpetic neuralgia
    pain 44
    prevention of 28
Postlaminectomy syndrome 64
Preservative free normal saline 28, 57
Procedural kit 3*f*
Proctalgia fugax 50
Provocative lumbar discography 71
Pterygomaxillary fissure 18*f*, 20
Pterygopalatine fossa 18*f*, 19*f*
Pudendal nerve block 4, 7, 54, 55*f*

R

Radiation enteritis 50
Radiofrequency ablation 7, 25, 25*f*, 27, 27*f*,
    40, 41*f*, 42, 68, 69
Rectal tenesmus 50
Rectum 50

Respiratory failure 35
Rib fractures 44
Rivaroxaban 9
Ropivacaine 10

S

Sacral hiatus 66*f*
Sacroiliac joint 79*f*
    injection 7, 78, 79*f*, 80*f*
Sacrum, sacral promontory point of 51*f*
Scoliosis 2
Shoulder
    osteoarthritis 35
    pain 35
Sphenopalatine ganglion 4
    block 6, 19, 19*f*, 20*f*
Spinal cord 24*f*
    infarct 32, 43, 56, 58, 60, 62, 63
    injury 43
    stimulator 7, 33*f*
        trial 5, 32, 73, 75*f*, 76*f*
Spinal needle 4*f*
    advance 17, 55, 63, 66, 69, 79
Spinous tubercles 81*f*
Splanchnic nerve block 4, 45, 45*f*, 46*f*
Standard epidural steroid injection 28, 56, 58, 60
Stellate ganglion 4, 6
    block 34
Steroid 11, 35
    sparing 32, 84, 87
Stocker's formula 3
Sufentanil 77
Superior articular process 25, 29, 39, 42, 51, 58
Superior hypogastric plexus 4
    block 7, 50, 51*f*, 52*f*

T

Tachycardia 11
Target anterior inferior iliac spine 86*f*
Temporomandibular joint injection 6
Testicular cancer pain 50
Third occipital nerve 7, 24, 26*f*, 27
    block 27
Thoracic
    epidural steroid injection 6, 42

facet intra-articular injection 6, 38*f*, 39*f*
interlaminar epidural steroid injection 42*f*, 43*f*
intra-articular facet injection 38
medial branch
    anatomic location of 41*f*
    block 40, 40*f*, 41
neuropathic pain 44
spondylosis 38, 40
Ticagrelor 9
Total spinal block 15
Transcrural technique 7, 47
Transforaminal epidural steroid injection 4, 7, 11
Trapezoids, midpoint of 27*f*
Triamcinolone acetonide 12
Trigeminal nerve 4, 18
    distribution 15
Trigeminal neuralgia 15
Tuohy needle, advance 58

U

Upper neck pain 24

V

Ventral laminar margin 29*f*
Vertebral
    artery 24*f*
    body 27, 29, 39
        anterior portion of 83*f*
    margin, anterolateral margin of 47*f*

W

Worsening
    headache 15
    pain 32, 43, 56, 58, 60, 62, 63

X

X-ray
    generator 1
    tube 1
Xylocaine 10

Z

Ziconotide 77